The Customer Oriented Laboratory

Practical Laboratory Management Series

The Customer Oriented Laboratory

William O. Umiker, MD
Adjunct Professor of Clinical Pathology
Hershey Medical Center
Penn State University
Hershey, Pennsylvania

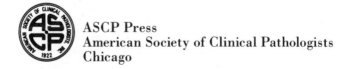

ASCP Press
American Society of Clinical Pathologists
Chicago

Acquisition and Development: Joshua Weikersheimer
Editor: Stephen Borysewicz
Production Manager: Lisa Pollak
Production Coordinator: Jennifer Sabella

Printed on Recycled Paper ♻

Other Volumes in the Practical Laboratory Management Series:
Volume I: Developing Performance Standards for Hospital Personnel

Library of Congress Cataloging-in-Publication Data

Umiker, William O.
   The customer-oriented laboratory / William O. Umiker.
      p. 200   — (Practical laboratory management series)
   Includes bibliographical references and index.
   ISBN 0-89189-310-5
   1. Medical laboratories — Quality control. 2. Medical
laboratories — Management.   I. Title.   II. Series.
   [DNLM: 1. Consumer Satisfaction — standards. 2. Laboratories —
organization & administration.   3. Laboratories — standards.   QY 23
U495c]
RB36.3.Q34U47   1991
362.1'77 — dc20
DNLM/DLC
for Library of Congress   90-14562
                                                                                CIP

Printed in the United States of America.

94   92   93   91   4   3   2   1

This book is dedicated to the following Sisters of St. Francis of Philadelphia who taught me what "caring" really means: Sr. Maria Dolorata Sullivan, Sr. Suzanne Marie Evans, Sr. Joan Dreisbach, and Sr. Margaret Aloysius McGrail.

Contents

Preface

Clinical laboratories have consistently led the charge toward the goal of quality excellence. They have moved from quality control (QC) to quality assurance (QA). As quality assurance matures into total quality management (TQM) or total quality improvement (TQI), the word customer or client appears with increasing regularity. In their broadest meanings; QA, TQM and TQI can be defined as "meeting or exceeding all of the expectations of all the clients."

Everything from the hiring of employees to the readability of lab reports determines how well clients are served.

This book presents concepts and practical applications that assist laboratorians at all hierarchical levels in meeting the challenge of satisfying all categories of customers.

We start by identifying all the laboratory clients, determining their expectations, designing and implementing in-service educational programs, and adopting a multiple participating group strategy.

The remaining chapters provide detailed information and practical suggestions on the use of special skills and techniques for implementing the changes needed to effect a comprehensive client-oriented service.

1. Who Are Our Customers and What Do They Want?

CUSTOMERS ARE THE recipients of our services. There are external and internal customers.

A customer is not an interruption of our work . . . he or she is the purpose of it.

EXTERNAL CUSTOMERS

Patients are principal end users of our services, but while the average inpatient has contact with about 50 people per admission, there is little or no direct contact with laboratorians.

The typical patient judges the quality of laboratory service by the technical and interpersonal skills of phlebotomists, the courtesy of the clerical staff, and the promptness with which billing questions are answered.[1]

Physicians enjoy a preferred customer status. Laboratory service manuals reflect this. Physicians demand quality work, rapid turnaround time, 24-hour availability, expert laboratory consultations, and reports that are prompt and easy to interpret.

Third-party payers, the people who pay the bills are customers, as are physicians' office staffs, freestanding outpatient facilities, and blood donors.

"It's not the employer who pays wages. He only handles the money. It's the customer who pays the wages." (Henry Ford)

Internal Customers

Because nurses do not prescribe tests, they are often overlooked as customers. Nevertheless, many of their duties are impacted by laboratory services. When delayed

1

or lost reports prevent nurses from administering the next dose of medication, they respond with the same vehemence as retail customers who have been ignored.

If instructions for collecting specimens are unclear the laboratory usually hears about it first from a nurse. Nurses' needs include transportation of specimens, information on specimen requirements, instructions for patient preparation for testing, and laboratory reports that are ready for attending physicians.

Administrators are served by all departments and therefore may be classified as customers. Executives are content when operational costs are kept at a minimum, and complaints are not forthcoming from any other customers.

Other departments are customers. Every individual or group who receives reports from the laboratory is a customer. This includes surgical review, infection control, and transfusion committees, and departments such as finance, human resources, and planning.

Laboratories, in turn, are served by departments such as human resources, materials management, and housekeeping. All too often these departments fail to realize that the laboratory is a client. A little problem, such as no cookies from the dietary service when blood donor hours commence, can provoke angry dialogues.

If you operate a school of medical technology, are not the recipients of your teaching efforts your customers? Is not each instructor a provider?

As recipients of our managerial expertise, our employees are also clients. They have individual and collective needs and preferences that should be actively solicited.

WHAT DO CUSTOMERS WANT?

"Give them what they want. Better still, give them more than they're used to."[2]

Consumers complain about the incompetency and discourtesy of service providers. Supermarket checkers mumble a robotic "thank you," or "have a nice day" because this is demanded of them by their employers. This is the simplest but least effective attempt at courteous customer service. Even when courtesy seems sincere and enthusiastic, incompetence may persist. A phlebotomist may introduce himself with a big smile, but put the blood specimen in the wrong tubes. A laboratory receptionist may exude friendliness, but can not answer simple questions about the scheduled procedure. Patients want a pleasant environment, good outcomes and caring, competent employees. More specifically, patients want us to:

1. be prepared and informed
2. be competent
3. be well groomed
4. have ready the necessary equipment and supplies
5. make them feel important and not patronize them
6. be courteous, friendly, and caring; show concern and ask questions
7. listen and respond to their feelings, and apologize and acknowledge appropriately
8. follow up (deliver on our promises)

Following is a list of ten specifics that physicians want from us.[3]

1. an adequate test menu
2. information about tests
3. information about patient preparation
4. appropriate specimens
5. skillful and courteous phlebotomy
6. quality procedures
7. rapid turnaround time
8. reports that are easy to read and interpret
9. readily available useful consultations
10. reasonable cost

Who is responsible for customer service? Every employee is!!!!

Guest relations

Guest relations is the strategy that seeks to redefine employee-customer interactions. Patients are treated as if they are a guest in the employee's home. Included as "guests" are other employees, physicians, and customers such as visitors and family members.[4] In other words, guest relations is nothing more than good customer service.

How employers and service providers benefit from good service

Benefits to Employers

Good service retains customers. According to the International Customer Service Institute, attracting a new customer costs five times as much as maintaining a current one.[2]

Benefits to Employees

"A company that sees customer service as important for all of its employees will almost always have the most productive and psychologically healthy environment."[5]

Good feelings are carried over to employees' personal lives.
Stress and frustration are reduced.
Needed improvements are identified.
Good relationships are established.
Patience and understanding from customers are obtained for the future.
Self-confidence is strengthened.
There is a possible increase in rewards (merit pay, promotion, or recognition, and job security).

Customer Complaint Form

Date:

Person recording incident:

Customer reporting incident:

Customer category (patient, nurse, physician etc):

Description of incident (what, where, when, and who):

How was incident handled and by whom?

How can this be prevented or handled better in the future?

Comments by responsible supervisor:

Signature of Lab Director:

Figure 1.1   A simple customer complaint form.

CUSTOMER-ORIENTED QUALITY

Laboratory customer-oriented quality relates to the flow of work. This begins with requests for service—the input—and ends with a report.

Customer-oriented quality addresses customer expectations rather than the expectations of the Joint Commission on Accreditation of Healthcare Organizations (JCAHO) and other accrediting agencies. In fact, the JCAHO now recognizes this need. Its 1990 standards include the requirement of a process for patient feedback and response.[6] Customer-oriented quality involves all aspects of work and all personnel.

Take a second look at your department. Then ask yourself these questions:

Is our laboratory, like many airlines and municipal agencies, characterized by the dogged pursuit of mediocrity?
Do we depend on a convenient location or captive customers?
Do we know who our customers are and what they want?
Are we making a serious and continuous effort to improve?
Do we see service as a challenge or do we regard customers as inconveniences?
Do we occasionally discuss ethical considerations?

Feedback Methodology and Sources

"We must learn how to listen to customers. And then we must help them identify and articulate their needs."[7]

A client feedback strategy should answer these questions:

Have we overlooked any client category?
Are there additional services we should offer now?
Are there additional services we should offer later?
How good is our service?
In relation to our competitors, what are our strengths, weaknesses, opportunities, and threats?

Include client participation during planning and provision of a new service. If you give clients a chance, they will do your market research for you.[8] Incident reports and complaints can be used to obtain customer feedback. Work at being approachable. Make it easy for clients to register complaints, ask questions, or make suggestions. Complaints should be recorded in a separate file and reviewed periodically. There should be a comparable method for collecting and publicizing positive feedback. An example of a simple customer complaint or commendation form is shown in Figure 1.1. An absence of unsolicited complaints does not necessarily mean that your clients are satisfied.

Formal studies based on periodic surveys, which are usually mailed in, are also important. Each customer group should be sampled. Do not forget your employees as both customers and providers. Employees are closest to the clients and spot problems first. An example of such a periodic survey form is shown in Figure 1.2.[9]

Data should be gathered at the time, or shortly after, a service is provided. These may be obtained through written questionnaires face-to-face or telephone interviews. Examples you are familiar with include hotel questionnaires for guests and follow-up calls after automobile service. Laboratories may easily use this method to evaluate phlebotomy or blood donor service.[10] An advantage of this strategy is that the personnel know that each client will have an opportunity to evaluate their performance.

Focus groups, such as wine and cheese meetings for physicians' office staffs, can be very worthwhile. Committee reports (transfusion, quality assurance, or utilization) provide updates. Laboratory or institutional sales representatives can obtain information from physician-clients about your service and that of your competitors. Patients' representatives or risk managers and key laboratory specialists who visit selected clients, eg, clinic laboratories, are good sources. Feedback is also returned from daily interactions between staff and clients. "Frequent and meaningful communication with physicians and other consumers facilitates the flow of pertinent and timely information needed to provide a better . . . service."[7]

When staff members are sensitized to the need for feedback, they solicit comments from the clients, who then become "coinvestigators." Keep asking "How can we improve this service?" Ask this in the hallways, in the doctors'

Client satisfaction questionnaire
Laboratory service evaluation
Your professional opinion is vitally important to us and we want to know how you feel about our laboratory services.

Importance of service

	Very Important	Important	Somewhat Important	Not Important

How do you rate our overall services?

1. Turnaround time ☐ ☐ ☐ ☐
2. Quality (reliability of results) ☐ ☐ ☐ ☐
3. Pricing (competitive fees) ☐ ☐ ☐ ☐
4. Stat service ☐ ☐ ☐ ☐
5. Critical abnormals called ☐ ☐ ☐ ☐
6. Courier services ☐ ☐ ☐ ☐
7. Supplies provided ☐ ☐ ☐ ☐
8. Patient handling ☐ ☐ ☐ ☐
9. Pathology services ☐ ☐ ☐ ☐
10. Client relations/customer service ☐ ☐ ☐ ☐
11. Billing ☐ ☐ ☐ ☐
12. Communication (information) ☐ ☐ ☐ ☐
13. Courtesy (employees) ☐ ☐ ☐ ☐
14. Call-backs ☐ ☐ ☐ ☐
15. Telephone etiquette ☐ ☐ ☐ ☐
16. Test mix (available tests) ☐ ☐ ☐ ☐
17. Convenience (locations) ☐ ☐ ☐ ☐
18. Requisition form ☐ ☐ ☐ ☐
19. Report format ☐ ☐ ☐ ☐
20. Caring attitude ☐ ☐ ☐ ☐

How do you rate our diagnostic services?

1. Profiles ☐ ☐ ☐ ☐
2. Chemistry ☐ ☐ ☐ ☐
3. Immunology ☐ ☐ ☐ ☐

11. Histology ☐ ☐ ☐ ☐
12. Blood Bank ☐ ☐ ☐ ☐

What do you like most about us? _____
What do you like least about us? _____
How could we improve service to you? _____

How did you choose us? ☐ **Referred** ☐ **Our sales representative**
☐ **Yellow Pages** ☐ **Location** ☐ **Word of mouth** ☐ **Direct mail**
☐ **Personal contact** ☐ **Contract with third party** ☐ **Bid** ☐ **Other** _____
Comments/Suggestions _____

Figure 1.2 Client satisfaction questionnaire. (Reprinted, by permission, from Fantus JA: A guide to marketing your lab's service: Laying the groundwork. *MLO* 1987;19:39–45.)

How well we perform

Excellent	Good	Fair	Poor	Does not apply
☐	☐	☐	☐	☐
☐	☐	☐	☐	☐
☐	☐	☐	☐	☐
☐	☐	☐	☐	☐
☐	☐	☐	☐	☐
☐	☐	☐	☐	☐
☐	☐	☐	☐	☐
☐	☐	☐	☐	☐
☐	☐	☐	☐	☐
☐	☐	☐	☐	☐
☐	☐	☐	☐	☐
☐	☐	☐	☐	☐
☐	☐	☐	☐	☐
☐	☐	☐	☐	☐
☐	☐	☐	☐	☐
☐	☐	☐	☐	☐
☐	☐	☐	☐	☐
☐	☐	☐	☐	☐
☐	☐	☐	☐	☐
☐	☐	☐	☐	☐
☐	☐	☐	☐	☐
☐	☐	☐	☐	☐
☐	☐	☐	☐	☐

lounge, and at social events. Periodically "dial-a-doc" and pop the question. Contact new physician-clients after they have used your service for a few weeks. Ask how things are going and how your service compares with what they had before. Supervisors should observe directly, by accompanying phlebotomists, relocating their desks to strategic points, and practicing *managing-by-walking-around.* Also arrange for cross-departmental meetings.

Employees should be solicited by periodic attitude surveys, as well as day-to-day personal contacts.[11] Even better are formal employees' appraisals of their leaders' performance. These "reverse performance appraisals" are usually elicited via anonymous questionnaires. The survey information is used to develop individual remedial educational programs for the managers, and to reward superior supervisory service.

When employees are permitted to rate their managers, leadership problems can be identified before serious hurt has been inflicted. Sexual harassment, favoritism, discrimination and intolerable autocratic leadership may be averted or stopped.[5]

Whatever the feedback channel, get the results, good or bad, to the appropriate people as soon as possible. Help them develop remedial measures if necessary.

Invalid Excuses for not Getting Feedback

"We don't have the time."
"We seldom get complaints."
"You can never satisfy our customers."
"They will only expect still better service."
"Frankly, I'm afraid that what we learn will discourage our staff."
"There's really nothing more we could do."

REFERENCES

1. Maratea JM: What ever happened to service? *MLO* 1988;20:19.

2. Peters T: *Surviving on Chaos: Handbook for a Management Revolution.* New York, Alfred A. Knopf, 1988.

3. Statland BE: Quality management: Watchword for the '90s. *MLO* 1989; 21:33–49.

4. Sage DR, Stahl MB: Creating a more caring work environment. *Manage Sol* 1987;32:5–14.

5. Bernstein AJ, Rozen SC: *Dinosaur Brains: Dealing With All Those Impossible People at Work.* New York, John Wiley & Sons, 1989.

6. *Accreditation Manual.* Chicago, Joint Commission on Accreditation of Healthcare Organizations, 1990, p 21.

7. Martin BG: 11 keys to quality management in the lab. *MLO* 1990;22:46–47.

8. Goldzimer L: *'I'm First': Your Customer's Message to You*. New York, Rawson Associates, 1989.

9. Fantus JA: A guide to marketing your lab's service: Laying the groundwork. *MLO* 1987;19:39–45.

10. Q&A. *MLO* 1989;21:77.

11. MacStravic RES: A new role-and-feedback system for the supervisor and the organization. *Health Care Super* 1990;8:23–34.

2. Planning Your New Program

A SAILOR LEANING OVER the rail of his ship was told that the ship was on fire. "So what?" he responded, "It's not my ship." A client-oriented attitude is achieved when every laboratory employee understands that good service is expected, that exceptional service will be rewarded, and that bad service will not be tolerated.

Leaders' words and deeds are the touchstones of a service ethos that shapes employee behavior. Leaders nurture this ethos by communicating values, becoming personally involved in service activities, and backing up slogans with actions. They demonstrate their belief in this new value system by treating their employees as they want employees to treat customers.[1]

THE THEORY OF CONTINUOUS IMPROVEMENT

Gone are the days when hospitals and laboratories could afford to be technology driven without explicit consideration of their customers' concerns. State-of-the-art technology alone does not meet these customers' needs.

Continuous improvement in service is our imperative. The needs and expectations of clients are constantly changing. This demands a perpetually willing attitude on the part of service providers who want to be on the cutting edge of customer satisfaction.

Managers, supervisors, patient representatives, quality assurance coordinators, and cost-control reviewers cannot improve customer service by themselves. Every provider must get into the act. The "Theory of Continuous Improvement" works only when it is pervasive.

SERVICE STRATEGY

Our service strategy is a special prescription that meets all the needs and exceeds all the expectations of our clients. It represents a two-pronged approach: "high-tech" and "high-touch." It anticipates customer needs by keeping in close touch with those customers.

Services originate as a vision. The vision is translated into a mission statement, goals are enunciated, and action plans are constructed.

Leaders have vision, managers have plans.

Mission statements must:

not be euphemistic hot air.
not be limited to the work itself. They must include what is done for clients.
reflect the core purpose of the department.
go beyond the work itself to include what is being accomplished for others.
be linked to visible actions that are obvious to all.

Short statements have greater impact and are remembered better. One word, such as *kaizen*, (a Japanese word meaning "never-ending quest for perfection") may do the trick.[2]

Following is an example of a laboratory mission statement:

"We're committed to listen to our customers, to establish appropriate standards, and to meet or exceed these specifications."[3]

STRATEGIC PLANNING

Strategic planning starts with market research. Market research information can be demographic or psychographic.[4] Demographic information relates to factors such as age, home location, education, income bracket, and family size. Psychographic information concerns preferences, expectations, attitudes, and other intellectual data.[4] An example of a psychographic needs analysis is shown in Figure 2.1. Similar data can be obtained from any of the sources listed in Chapter 1.

The next step in strategic planning is to formulate goals. These should be written rather than merely stated, because studies have shown that written goals are much more likely to be achieved. The projected goal takes form when everyone can visualize and take pride in the ultimate outcome of the program. Targets become more specific when goals are subdivided into objectives. Consider the following example:

Goal: to improve outpatient satisfaction with blood collection.
Objectives: 1. relocate phlebotomy station by (date).
             2. offer evening hours by (date).
             3. provide 10 hours of special instruction to phlebotomists by (date).

Service Activity: Outpatient phlebotomy station

Subdivisions of Service	Customer Ratings (n = 100)
Available hours	Fair
Parking facilities	Good
Convenience of location of station	
Ambulatory	Good
Physically handicapped	Poor
Comfort of waiting area	Great
Length of wait	Good
Courtesy of receptionist	Fair
Explanation of charges	Poor
Courtesy of phlebotomists	Great
Skill of phlebotomists	Great

Improvement Needs Perceived by Patients:

1. Available hours: Twenty responders would like evening hours. Five patients want 0700–0800 hours so they can get served before going to work.

2. Convenience: Patients with ambulatory restrictions find the walk from the hospital entrance to the station difficult.

3. Courtesy: One receptionist is curt and impatient. None seem well informed about charges and billing practices.

Positive patient comments:
Many patients commented on the courtesy and skill of most of the phlebotomists. They compared our service favorably with that of competitors.

Figure 2.1   Example of a market research survey.

Customer-Oriented Approach

Our plan encompasses the following activities:

1. Hire employees who are client-oriented as well as technically or professionally competent.
2. Provide an orientation and training program that stresses client satisfaction.
3. Anticipate changes in customers' needs or expectations and monitor their satisfaction by using multiple feedback sources and techniques.
4. Encourage all employees to participate in the planning and execution of new or improved services, as well as in solving customer problems.
5. Provide an intensive continuing education program that features client satisfaction.

CHANGES IN THE INFRASTRUCTURE AND STAFFING

The largest cost of producing great service is that of creating infrastructures — networks of people, physical facilities, instrumentation, and information that support the production of client service. Technological changes constantly threaten to render existing infrastructures obsolete and inefficient.[1]

These changes should be based on what is best for clients, not for the convenience of the staff. A common violation of this principle is the staffing of evening shifts by the least experienced employees, and the filling of weekend slots with part-time employees who lack the competency of the weekday workers.

Client Representatives

Some hospitals already have patient representatives, or "ombudsmen." Risk managers also function as patient representatives. These people smooth ruffled feathers and prevent complaints from becoming formal grievances or lawsuits.[5]

Employees, as clients, may have union or nonunion representation. Officers of the medical staff look out for the interests of their members. The financial interests of third-party payers are addressed by utilization review committees, peer review organizations, and representatives of medical insurance companies. While the Joint Commission on Accreditation of Healthcare Organizations (JCAHO) is not a customer, hospitals spend more time and money trying to satisfy the quality assurance demands of that organization than they commit to satisfying known and knowable improvement demands of customers.

Consider the Following Special Assignments

1. Patient-service representative. I do not recommend this for most laboratories because client interest should be everyone's responsibility. However, in large laboratories it may be desirable to funnel complaints through one specially trained person.
2. Nursing service coordinator. Weekly visits to nursing stations by a laboratory representative who discusses nursing-laboratory problems can result in better usage of laboratory service, and better interdepartmental relationships.[6]
3. Technical director or educator in charge of the overall in-service educational activities for your improved customer service program.
4. Chairpersons or facilitators for special committees or quality circles.

ADMINISTRATIVE ACTIONS

Three kinds of administrative actions (changes) can result in better customer service: structural, procedural and behavioral.[7]

A *structural change* may be relocation of the outpatient phlebotomy room, creation of a special parking area for blood donors, updating of the laboratory information system, or installation of a better automatic analyzer.

A *procedural change* (how we do things) is usually dictated by a policy. For example, outpatient satisfaction may be enhanced by changing the hours that the phlebotomy station is open.

Take a second look at your policies. Review your policy and procedure manual. Evaluate each item from a customer's standpoint. Determine if it augments or inhibits customer service. If these policies are recorded on a word processor, your task is easy. Simply use the "select" mode to focus on statements that include the names of client categories: patient, physician, nurse, etc. Expurgate or revise policies or procedures that have a negative effect.

Scrutinize each new policy or procedure that is proposed. Introduce additional policies or procedures needed to improve client service, such as home blood specimen collection, or teaching patients the use of self-diagnostic kits.

Among the most important policies are those dealing with hiring practices, orientation of new employees, position descriptions, work standards, and performance appraisals. These should be revised with the customer in mind. The McDonnell-Douglas Corp promulgated the following nine policies[8]:

1. Careful assessment of candidates.
2. Revised orientation to instill corporate values.
3. Challenging assignments.
4. 40 hours of training per employee.
5. Coaching and mentoring.
6. Annual career counseling sessions.
7. Emphasis on performance evaluations.
8. Pay-for-performance.
9. Duty change every 7 years.

Construct a policy regarding the registration, investigation, and resolution of incident reports and complaints (now mandated by the JCAHO). Record these in a separate file and review them periodically (see Figure 1.2). Do not neglect a comparable method for collecting and publicizing positive feedback.

Establish a well-publicized channel for inviting suggestions and introducing new techniques or procedures from all your customers, especially your employees. Do not rely on suggestion boxes. Focus groups, questionnaires, and staff meetings are all appropriate.

Behavioral change in service people is often more difficult to bring about. It takes convincing, training, and coaching. Select the right employees and orient them well.

The Reward System

The extra effort in selecting and indoctrinating will be love's labor lost if the desired behavior is not rewarded. Rewards should remind people of the mission statement.

What gets done is what gets rewarded.

Using position descriptions and work expectations as standards, revise performance rating systems to include customer satisfaction. These changes are doubly effective if pay-for-performance systems are in place.

Rewards should be monetary when possible, but the reward program should be as comprehensive as possible. Nonmonetary rewards include praise, recognition, formal and informal ceremonies, rituals, and celebrations. While promotions may not be readily available, the star performers can be given time off, special trips, inexpensive tokens of appreciation, and opportunities to expand their expertise and to enhance their careers.

Performance appraisals provide ideal opportunities to express your satisfaction with the client-service aspect of employee behavior. The planning segment of these reviews should include discussions of better customer quality, and the melding of client satisfaction into each employee's new goals and objectives.

Monitoring Performance

Direct observations by supervisors are of utmost importance. First-line supervisors are the managers who are closest to the daily employee-client interactions. They can become the most effective customer-service representatives.

The recording of "critical" incidents, good and bad, is an essential component of an effective performance appraisal system. The work of marginal performers must be closely monitored; feedback should be obtained frequently from the recipients of their services. This includes documentation of complaints, and the use of customer surveys.

Receptionists and office personnel usually exhibit impeccable courtesy, but professionals and laboratory assistants who answer the telephone, or who give out verbal reports, may be tactless or downright discourteous. Some employees treat customers as nuisances rather than clients. When supervisors overhear rude telephone responses and fail to admonish the offending employee, they are neglecting an important responsibility.

Supervisors who spend all of their time in their offices simply can not monitor service. Japanese employers are well aware of this, and position their managers right in the middle of the production areas. Enclosed offices are anathema to the Japanese.

Managing by walking around is highly recommended. It is essential to active leadership. Managers who are responsible for those employees who provide patient services directly must make a special monitoring effort. This means periodically accompanying phlebotomists on their daily rounds, spending some time in the outpatient blood-collection units, and listening to telephone dialogues.

Financial Resources

Increased funding may be necessary for service-related items such as computers, pneumatic tube systems, renovations, and equipment that improve the speed or quality of service.

Selecting the best instruments and procedures can cut costs, reduce turnaround time, or improve accuracy. This benefits patients, physicians, nurses, and third-party payers. Cole[9] found that selecting the best instruments and test profiles yielded increased productivity, decreased "stat" requests, and shorter turnaround.

Communication

Formal and informal channels of communication transmit customer-related information constantly. Make a list of client categories (patient, physician) and with these document how communication is maintained. Look for ways to improve communication.

Most laboratories have a newsletter for physicians and nurses that provides information relating to new tests, better specimen handling, and report interpretation.

Intralaboratory bulletins feature new procedures, progress, or QA reports, and special reports from laboratory sections, committees, and quality-service groups.

REFERENCES

1. Davidow WH, and Uttal B: *Total Customer Service: The Ultimate Weapon.* New York, Harper & Row, 1989.
2. Peters T: *Thriving on Chaos.* New York, Alfred A Knopf, 1988.
3. Statland BE: Quality management: Watchword for the '90s. *MLO* 1989;21:33–40.
4. Albrecht K, Zemke R: *Service America: Doing Business in the New Economy.* Homewood, Ill, Dow-Jones-Irwin, 1985.
5. Buckout CH: Marketing the hospital through guest relations. *Hosp Admin Curr* 1987;31:7–12.
6. Umiker W: Troubleshooting lab-nursing service problems. *MLO* 1983;15:80–86.
7. Day CM: Three diagnostic clues to management problems. *MLO* 1987;19:74–79.
8. Settle M: Up through the ranks at McDonnell Douglas. *Personnel* 1989;66:17–22.
9. Cole GW: Improving lab utilization through test profiles. *MLO* 1982;14:32–38.

3. In-Service Educational Programs

CUSTOMER-ORIENTED QUALITY begins and ends with education. The first two legs of our strategy were operational planning and administrative actions. The third is developing an in-service program. Japanese business professionals are particularly cognizant of the importance of worker education; up to 20% of workers' time in Japanese-owned US plants is spent in training.[1] Technical and professional training is essential. If employees lack the knowledge and skill to perform competently, any customer-service program will be nothing more than window dressing. Such unfortunate workers are like teachers who are expert in the essentials of education but do not know their subject material.

Another potential weakness is that of considering the needs only of external customers, and ignoring internal clients. For example, a pathologist may be active in the College of American Pathologists, and neglect his pathology residents.

"Why do some employees know exactly what to do, while others don't? It's all in how you train and manage them."[2]

In our educational program, some client service topics are important to all laboratory members. As many employees as possible should attend sessions that deal with these topics. Special programs are selected for employees who have direct contact with clients. These "customer contact agents" include phlebotomists, receptionists, supervisors, employees who serve blood donors, and those who use the telephone often.

Planning must be thorough because large chunks of time are expended in any comprehensive educational effort. Around-the-clock staffing and high turnover rates necessitate repetition of each educational offering.

CHANGING BEHAVIOR OF PERSONNEL

The Importance of Persuasion

Persuasiveness is important because established behavioral patterns are not easy to change. Lucy, a 20-year veteran of laboratory-nursing wars, is not ready to accept nurses as laboratory clients. Lucy, and others, labeled as "change-resistant," do not really resist change. They resist the manner in which the change is introduced.[3] Persuasion is achieved when employees see *why* change is needed, and they have input into the *what* and the *how* of the change. The most persuasive presenters are those who have earned the respect of the participants.

While outside motivational speakers can kick off a new program, supervisors are the key persons in any sustained program. Supervisors are the behavioral models, the formal and informal trainers, and they provide the crucial orientation of new employees. They reinforce or erode what employees learn at training sessions. Without their input, the educational program may amount to nothing more than "smile at client" sessions.

Meetings must be practical and palatable to participants. Learning experiences are enhanced if audience participation is vigorous and the talks are freewheeling. Seminars and workshops provide formal approaches. Videotapes or audiotapes of these meetings may be worthwhile. When presenters and facilitators know that they are being recorded, they prepare more thoroughly, and presentations are honed to excellence. These tapes can be shown to orientees as well as to employees who miss the original presentations.

Commercially obtained audiotapes and videotapes can be quite worthwhile. They ensure quality training and standardized practices, and they can save time. The award-winning ASCP videotape *Blood Collection: The Routine Venipuncture* is a prime example. It features a step-by-step demonstration of actual venipuncture and emphasizes patient rapport, accuracy, and safety. In most laboratories the turnover of phlebotomists places a heavy burden on trainers. Such an educational tool can lighten that burden.

Large organizations may use payroll inserts to remind employees that their work attitudes make a difference in customer service. Employees read them because they are brief. They pay attention to them because they make sense.

The most effective social training is informal, whether in groups or one-on-one. The buddy system is very effective as long as the senior buddy has the right attitude and behavior.

Learning experiences are reinforced when supervisors support the behavioral changes discussed at these meetings, and serve as exemplars. A good way to get off to a bad start is for the senior lab members to show up only for the first one or two sessions.

"There is no teaching to compare with example." (Robert Baden Powell)

The first session of our educational program provides a general introduction. It focuses on the subjects described earlier—customer identification, client satisfaction, mission statements, goals, and the agenda for the educational program. This session is critical. Success or failure hinges on whether or not the employees buy into the program.

Team Building is a Major Educational Goal

Morale is higher and turnover lower in closely knit groups.

Teamwork must be based on commitment to the customer and to constant improvement.[4] It refers to a spirit of loyalty and collegiality, and results from a common understanding of the laboratory's vision and values.[2] The "turned-on team" is there 100% of the time, physically and mentally. Its members have a sense of self-confidence. They like having problems to solve, and they feel a sense of power.[5]

Effective team members have a clear vision of departmental goals and objectives. They have an all-consuming passion for quality. They set quality goals for themselves and break down barriers to quality performance, be they policies, procedures, physical factors, or people. Team members comprehend how their productivity and competency affect customer service, they feel they have control over how they do their work, and they have input into problem solving and troubleshooting.

The two key elements of team leadership are structure and function. The structure includes the policies, procedures, and expectations that delineate a manager's accountability. Function concerns how the manager exercises these responsibilities, and shapes the work environment. The leader must serve as a model, provide challenge, and work with the team in formulating objectives and action plans.

Collaboration and participation are critical. Start by calling the members of your staff "associates," "colleagues," or "teammates"; avoid "subordinates." Make your people independent of you, but dependent on each other; employee *inter*dependence promotes teamwork.

Teamwork is promoted by group planning and goal setting. Goals should highlight customer and employee satisfaction. Articulate them in simple terms like these:

"to provide quick quality service"
"to create a great place to work"
"to give every employee an opportunity to be creative"
"to inculcate a sense of achievement"
"to move constantly in the direction of perfection"

Eleven Ways to Promote Teamwork

1. Increase the span of control. Industrial organizations promote teamwork by eliminating foremen and supervisors. Workers are divided into teams and leadership is shared or rotated. A less drastic strategy is simply to cut back the number of managers. The reduced availability of supervisors forces employees to depend more on one another.

2. Establish special work groups such as quality circles, committees, and task forces.
3. Develop "hybrid generalist-specialists." Job satisfaction increases when each employee in a work group is both a generalist and a specialist. As a generalist the person performs a variety of duties. This reduces monotony and increases group flexibility. As a specialist the individual's self-esteem is enhanced, and he or she is motivated to develop that specialization and to achieve self-actualization.
4. Cross train and rotate work stations.
5. Share leadership roles. The role of leader should shift with the problem at hand. Let the educational coordinator organize the training program, an associate pathologist develop and implement a quality assurance committee, and a senior phlebotomist head up a patient relations focus group.
6. Match each team member's strengths and interests to assigned tasks. Take advantage of strengths. Make weaknesses irrelevant.
7. Enhance participative management by encouraging social and recreational activities.
8. Keep communication channels buzzing via both formal and informal (grapevine) networks. Do not withhold bad news. When you are invited to a meeting, take a member of your team along.
9. Be willing to admit failures. Make each failure a learning situation. Encourage employees to stop thinking about who is right or wrong and consider what is right or wrong. [2]
10. Train, train, and train. Strike a balance between social and technical training.

Since you want each member of your group to be both a generalist and a specialist, a lot of training is necessary. Aim specifically at team-building by providing instruction in decision making and problem solving, listening and confrontational skills, and getting the most out of meetings.

11. Have lots of celebrations. Team effort must be fun, so a sense of humor is highly desirable. Celebrations demonstrate your interest in group accomplishments. The celebrations can consist of doughnuts and coffee, picnics, dinners, congratulatory letters, or awards of special insignia or trophies. Invite senior executives to some of the get-togethers.

Barriers to Teamwork

Threats of reductions-in-force
Competitive merit pay. Encourage team competition instead.
Conflict
Difficult or unproductive people
Absence of the positive factors already discussed.
(Note: Everyone should either lead or follow. There's no room for "deadwood" on a good team, so PRUNE IT.)

IN-SERVICE PROGRAMS FOR CUSTOMER CONTACT AGENTS

We want to augment the interactive skills of employees who have direct client contact. As previously stated, customer service is judged by the tact, cooperation, and communication skills of lab representatives — phlebotomists, receptionists, telephone communicators, blood donor personnel, and people who answer questions, give out reports, or address complaints.

A more personal service calls for healthy, deep-seated attitudes. Specific strategies may be required to nudge these attitudes in the right direction.

What Comes First, Attitude or Behavior?

We usually think of behavior as being responsive to attitudes, and that is frequently the case. But behavioral psychologists have shown that the reverse is often true: behavioral alterations can affect attitudes. You can get angry by frowning, feel better by smiling.

Experiments at the University of California demonstrated that simply placing a funny cartoon or a smiling caricature next to telephones evoked striking improvements in the phonetics of the employees who answered the telephone.[6] That is good news because changing attitudes directly is difficult since it means trying to get into other people's minds. It is much easier to direct behavior. The Marine Corps has proven this over and over. Marine officers do not try to change the attitudes of recruits. They learned long ago that if you got the men to behave like good Marines, their attitudes shaped up along with their bodies. So let us take a page from the Marines. We will adjust behavior, and not get involved with mind control.

Communications and Other Interactions

The appearance of personnel and facilities affects customers' judgement of the competency and caring of service providers. But while clean uniforms and background music are important, most caring comes from the quality of direct interactions between providers and clients.

Interactions include everything one says and does: facial expressions, touching, body language, explanation of the purpose of tests, and frequent use of the patient's name make for positive interactions. But, gossiping or arguing in front of patients, or appearing rushed or indifferent provoke negative reactions.[7]

The importance of these interactions has been beautifully described by Carlzon.[8] He took over a failing airline, SAS (Scandinavian Airlines System), and quickly made it successful and respected. He attributes much of his success to employees reacting to what he called "moments of truth." Each contact with a customer constitutes such a moment. For the average airline passenger there are only five such contacts per flight. For the average hospitalized patient there are about 50 such moments. Just one unpleasant encounter can undo what the other 49 accomplish.

Certain words can trigger emotional reactions from customers and must be avoided. Here are a few:

"No" without adequate explanation

"can't" Tell customers what you *can* do, not what you can't. Do not say: "I can't help you," or "That's not my responsibility."

"Policy" What they hear is that policy takes precedence over their needs.

Blaming the computer, "they," or someone other than "I" or "we".

Phlebotomists are Special

Blood collectors have more direct contact with patients than do most other laboratory employees. Their appearance, technical skill, and humanism are vital to the reputation of the laboratory. Phlebotomists are usually among the lowest paid members of the laboratory team, and often command little respect from nurses or laboratorians. Patients, not being fond of needle sticks, rarely greet blood collectors with welcoming smiles. Phlebotomists tire quickly of cliches like "not you again," or "here comes the vampire." These repetitive jolts to self-esteem partially account for the traditionally high turnover among phlebotomists.

These deprecatory factors can be reversed when phlebotomists get favorable feedback, intensive training, and assignments other than blood drawing, become eligible for certification, or receive minipromotions within their classification.[9] In one laboratory, comprehensive training plus a few pay increments improved the retention rate of its phlebotomists.[10]

REFERENCES

1. Maratea JM: What ever happened to service? *MLO* 1988;20:19.

2. Goldzimer LS: *'I'm First': Your Customer's Message to You*. New York, Rawson Associates, 1989.

3. Martin BG: 11 keys to quality management in the lab. *MLO* 1990;22:46–47.

4. Deming WE: *Quality, Productivity, and Competitive Position*. Cambridge, Mass, MIT Center for Advanced Engineering Study, 1982.

5. Kirby T: *The Can-do Manager*. New York, AMACOM Book Division, 1989.

6. Loehr JE, McLaughlin PJ: *Mentally Tough*. New York, E. Evans & Co, 1986.

7. MacStravic RS: A new role-and-feedback system. *Health Care Super* 1990;8:23–34.

8. Carlzon J: *Moments of Truth*. Cambridge, Mass, Ballinger Pub Co, 1987.

9. Golden T: The payoffs of a well-prepared phlebotomy team. *MLO* 1985;10:79–84.

10. Adams T, Menard C, Stevenson JW: Upgrading phlebotomy to cut employee turnover. *MLO* 1988;20:57–64.

4. Use of Employee Participating Groups

COMPREHENSIVE PROGRAMS REQUIRE what most of us have too little of—time. If delay is unavoidable or progress is slow, here is a simple interim strategy. At every meeting of every kind—committee, staff, budget, or planning—one member serves as client representative. These ombudsmen should be assertive individuals who do not hesitate to speak up and say "Wait a minute. That's not in the best interest of our clients," or "Tell us how that will benefit our patients," or "How will the nursing service react to that?" For maximum effectiveness, this role is rotated among the various group members.

In our quest for excellence in customer service we must have the cooperation of every laboratory employee. The more we can get these people involved in the planning process, the greater is the likelihood of motivating them in the workplace.

WHY SMALL GROUPS?

Most people function best in small groups. They have more individual control over the meeting process, they are more expressive when the number of members is limited, and they are comfortable with associates with whom they have daily close contact. In addition, small groups can focus on problems that involve every group member—there are no disinterested parties.

Depending exclusively on a quality assurance coordinator or customer-service representative will not do. From the employees' standpoint this just introduces another clipboard carrier who keeps them from getting their work done. The use of Employee Participating Groups (EPGs) is an effective type of decentralization. Delegating

23

to EPGs ensures that all employees who wish to, can get involved in analyzing, evaluating, and making recommendations for improving customer service.

As in the case of other forms of delegation, this powerful tool must be used skillfully. If a group suspects that it is being used only to increase productivity or to rubber-stamp policies from above, it will balk, just as will a delegate who feels that he or she is being dumped on.

Since EPGs involve team effort, in-service programs that emphasize teamwork and problem solving should precede the initiation of the group meetings. In a previous chapter, you read about team building. In this chapter and the two that follow, you will learn more about how effective groups function.

WHOM DO WE WANT IN OUR EPGS?

In the case of small laboratories, the team may consist of the entire staff. Some topics are best handled by individual laboratory sections or shifts, while activities that cross unit lines call for special committees or other EPGs. For example, consideration of a time-saving bacteriologic procedure is best discussed by the microbiology workers. On the other hand, analyses of request or reporting forms may be handled best by a special intersectional committee.

When possible and appropriate, invite special guests to some of these sessions. Such guests include clients, vendors, departmental or hospital members of the marketing department, and people from departments that serve or are served by the laboratory. Extend an open invitation to the hospital or laboratory sales representative who contacts physicians' offices, nursing homes, industrial firms, or other outside clients.

The specific names of the groups are less important than the process and content of the meetings. However, catchy titles such as *the cost-cutters* for a group investigating cost reductions; or *the front-enders* for a committee dealing with activities in the early phases of work flow, may have motivational impact.

Success of these groups depends on the enthusiasm of the members, the availability of sufficient time, and the amount of support provided by laboratory management. If recommendations are ignored or ridiculed, the program will quickly falter.

THAT MISSION STATEMENT AGAIN

At the first meeting of an EPG, the laboratory director should review the departmental mission statement, explain how the work of this group fits into the departmental strategy, and promise "open-door" availability to any member of the group who wants data or advice relating to current, past, or future topics.

The first order of business directed by the group leader is to construct a mission statement for the group. If members have difficulty articulating this, and most will, a simple approach is to respond to these key questions:

1. What is the goal of our group? This addresses the "what."
2. What is the purpose of this activity? This addresses the "why."

3. What strategy will we use? This addresses the "how."
4. (Optional) What is the bottom line? This describes the desired results.

Example: Mission Statement of a Hematology EPG

Goal

A hematology service that surpasses the expectations of our physician clients.

Purpose

To improve the quality of reported results, shorten turnaround, reduce costs, and promote a spirit of cooperation between members of the hematology staff, our clients, vendors, and fellow laboratorians in other sections.

Strategy

Meet weekly to analyze service needs, investigate complaints and suggestions, and explore new methods or equipment. Make recommendations to management. Monitor progress and evaluate results.

Bottom Line

Desired results include greater accuracy and precision, reduced turnaround time, lower costs, fewer complaints, and greater client satisfaction as determined by periodic customer surveys.

The above statements are easily synthesized into a concise mission statement. The fact that the group came up with this on its own has several benefits. (1) The members comprehend where they are going, and how they are going to get there. (2) Because they formulated the statement, their "ownership" ensures their support. (3) They have a sense of achievement. At their very first meeting they have accomplished something worthwhile.

What follows is a series of outlines of suggested topics for group action.

Group Action

Topic: Ethical Considerations

Clients: Patients, suppliers, third-party payers
Group: Committee of senior managers
Indicators:

Knowingly performing and billing for duplicate tests[1]
Assigning least experienced laboratorians to night shifts
Retaining an incompetent worker because he or she is a single parent and would have trouble finding a job[2]

Hiring only white phlebotomists because of unsupported belief that patients prefer white caregivers[2]

Disclosing confidential patient information[3]

Topic: Activities at "Front End" of Work Flow

Clients: Staff clinicians, nurses, physicians' office staff
Group: Committee or quality circle
Indicators:

Service manual
Menu of available services around the clock
Ease of requesting services, and obtaining products such as blood components
Availability of consultations
Ease of obtaining instructions for preparing patients or submitting specimens

Topic: Laboratory Utilization

Clients: Patients and third-party payers
Group: Utilization review committee
Indicators:

Physician ordering patterns
Indiscriminate stat orders; criteria may be over 15% of day shift, 35% on PM shift[1]
Timed orders
Demands for work to be completed and on charts by specific time
Late presurgical admissions

Note: Monitoring of laboratory utilization, principally overutilization and abuses, benefits not only the customers who pick up the tab, but also the patients who are not subjected to unnecessary or painful procedures.

Special focus should be on standing orders such as routine coagulation studies of preoperative patients, esoteric tests such as hormone assays, and high-cost and invasive tests such as bone marrow and fine-needle aspiration.[4]

Because the JCAHO's 1990 agenda calls for outcome-oriented quality assurance, greater attention will be paid to physician behaviors that affect lab costs. This requires data to show how physician ordering patterns influence test costs and case outcomes. Some 20% to 30% of tests are said to be unnecessary or inappropriate.[1]

Topic: Blood Specimen Collection

Clients: Patients and nurses
Group: Phlebotomists

Indicators:

Turnaround time
Safety techniques
Resticks
Courtesy toward patients
Explanations to patients and parents
Specimen sharing
Instruments that use smaller samples
Procedures that minimize repeat drawings[5]
Blood specimens collected on a 2-hour schedule rather than twice daily[6]
Use of a "specimen bank" to minimize repeat drawings[7]
Phlebotomy response time to intensive care units[4]

Topic: Activities at the "Back End" of Work Flow

Clients: Staff clinicians, nurses, physicians' office staff
Group: Special committee
Indicators:

Reporting of critical values
Stat and routine turnaround times
User-friendly report forms
Availability of telephone reports
Courtesy of reporting staff members
Quality of service
Value of pathologist's interpretations

Topic: Cost Control

Clients: Patients and third-party payers
Group: Finance committee
Indicators:

Internal data: costs, revenue, productivity, personnel utilization[8]
External data: projected service expansion or reduction plans, changes in
    reimbursement patterns[8]
Inappropriate ordering by house staff

Topic: Complaints and Errors

Clients: Patients and clinicians
Group: Department, section, or shift
Indicators:

Error rate[9]
Evaluations by clients (surveys)
Incident reports and complaints

Topic: *Blood Donation*

Clients: Blood donors
Group: Donor center personnel
Indicators:

Donor hours
Waiting time
Recruitment
Parking
Reception area
Phlebotomy facilities
Percentage of reactions
Percentage of unsuccessful draws

Topic: *Physicians' Office Laboratories*

Clients: Patients, physicians and their staffs
Group: Special committee
Indicators:

Consultations
Quality Control
Service as reference lab
Troubleshooting
Communication problems

REFERENCES

1. Barros A: A question of professional ethics. *MLO* 1989;21:17–18.
2. Eliopoulos C: Customer relations in the health care setting. *Health Care Super* 1986;4:19–31.
3. Anderson GR: Ethical thinking and decision making for health care supervisors. *Health Care Super* 1987;5:1–12.
4. Sharp JW: Implementing hospital-wide laboratory QA. *MLO* 1989;21:35–42.
5. Kattan D: Are we drawing too much blood? *MLO* 1986;18:75–76.
6. Cole GW: Improving lab utilization through test profiles. *MLO* 1982;14:32–38.
7. Adams T, Menard C, Stevenson JW: Upgrading phlebotomy to cut employee turnover. *MLO* 1988;20:57–64.
8. Barros A: Financial management is more than monitoring a budget! *MLO* 1982;14:43–47.
9. *MLO* 1989;21:77.

5. Quality Circles

HE QUALITY CIRCLE (QC) concept was developed in Japan in 1962. By 1982 there were more than one million quality circles in Japan.[1] QCs became popular in the United States because (1) they had the prestigious Japanese label, (2) they promised immediate improvements in productivity and quality, and (3) they utilized a bottom-up participative philosophy espoused by certain behavioral psychologists. One study estimated that 90% of the Fortune 500 companies had introduced QCs into their organizations in the early 1980s.[2]

The health care industry followed suit. Hospitalwide circles were mandated,[3,4] nurses formed them,[5] and laboratories reported favorable results in a broad spectrum of applications.[6–10]

DEFINITION OF A QC

A QC consists of a small group of employees doing similar work who meet voluntarily on a regular basis to identify, analyze, and solve work problems relating directly or indirectly to quality, productivity, or cost. QCs exist in many hybrid forms, with names such as "employee participating groups," "self-managing work teams," and "quality assurance committees."

If QCs are to be more than encapsulated additions to suggestion boxes, managers must be willing to accept the QC as a process or system rather than a program.[1]

QCs promote teamwork, while suggestion systems promote competition. QCs do more than most suggestion systems. They can raise employee productivity, and they can reduce turnover, absenteeism, and lost time. By involving hourly employees in operational decision making, QCs represent organizational political reform.[1]

Thompson[1] suggests that QCs and suggestion systems should be complementary. He states that the potential conflict between the two systems can be avoided by automatically submitting all QC proposals to the suggestion system, and rewarding QCs on a higher scale than that used to reward individuals.[1]

Characteristics of a Typical QC

A QC consists of 4 to 15 employees, including a leader, and a facilitator or advisor. Membership is voluntary, and a first-line supervisor serves as leader unless the circle consists of supervisors or managers. Members receive training in decision-making, problem-solving, and communication skills. The circle usually meets 1 hour per week, during work hours, on institutional premises. It may or may not have authority to implement the changes it recommends.

Problems Addressed and Anticipated Results

Originally, subjects were limited to quality, production, or cost. Discussions of salaries, benefits, policies, personalities, or supervisory problems were forbidden. Those restrictions have been lifted in many American companies. Topics now may include safety, job structure, control mechanisms, and quality assurance. Even aesthetics of the work environment may be deemed an appropriate subject.[11]

In the clinical laboratory, QCs have successfully addressed work flow patterns, blood collection, specimen processing, holiday scheduling, structural planning, policy making, and inventory control.[6-10] Schwabbauer et al[12] found that the QC approach to a continuing education program was highly successful.

QCs have two major goals: improved task performance and enhanced quality of work environment. Customer satisfaction is impacted directly by the former, indirectly by the latter.

Results are both tangible and intangible. Tangible results can be measured by "hard data" such as costs, output, audits, and documented complaints. Intangible results, such as improved communication, a sense of ownership, and improved morale, are more difficult to measure. Employee attitude surveys, turnover rates, and attendance records may be used, but are less susceptible to statistical analysis. Admittedly, these observations may result not from the QCs per se, but from the "Hawthorne effect" (improved performance due to increased attention given to employees), or to some unidentified coincidental factor.[13]

Incentives

Whenever a change such as the introduction of QCs is proposed, people turn on "Channel WIIFM" (What's In It For Me?). While this question may not be articulated, it is always in the minds of the people who are affected, and should be answered. Extrinsic rewards such as bonuses and performance ratings can be motivating factors.

Intrinsic motivators include recognition and the opportunity to control one's work. Most employees prefer to solve work problems rather than to gripe about them . . . but there are exceptions, aren't there? When a QC first begins, intrinsic motivators are powerful, but this effect eventually wanes unless the employees receive financial rewards or special challenges, or their efforts have a positive influence on their daily work.

Competition between circles may be beneficial or harmful depending on how it is handled. At its best, it stimulates competing groups. At its worst, it stifles cooperation and creates ill will.[1]

The first step is to sell the concept. Always proceed from the top down. First, sell the idea to executive management and the union, then to middle management, and finally to employees. Training should follow the same sequence.[1]

Forming a steering committee is an early option after the concept has been approved. Similar functions can be fulfilled by an administrative staff committee. This committee solicits input from representatives of all employee levels and job functions about instituting QCs. Such data include employee attitude questionnaires and customer satisfaction surveys.[4] Before the groups begin, the steering committee or a senior facilitator collects baseline data to be used to measure results of the new system.

The committee may recommend an outside consultant to explain the concept, to help organize the program, and to train facilitators.

SPECIAL MEMBERS OF THE QC

Leaders

Leaders must be skilled in leading group discussions and problem-solving as well as being technically and professionally competent.

Facilitators

Special staff members serve as facilitators or advisers. They (1) ensure that the leader and members receive adequate training in QC activities, and put this to use, (2) monitor progress, (3) prevent the leader from dominating the circle, and (4) interrupt nonproductive deliberations or straying from the agenda.

A facilitator meets with the leader before and after each QC meeting. Monthly meetings between the facilitator and a member of upper management are recommended for monitoring feedback.[4]

Union Representative

If the organization has a union, it is imperative that it be included in the QC from the very beginning. If possible, a union member should be on the steering committee.[1]

Other potential members include representatives of vendors, customers, and members of other departments who impact the activities of the QC.

Training Requirements

QCs require particular behavior that may conflict with traditional patterns. Therefore, people need formal training in how to fill their roles as leaders, facilitators, and members.

Facilitators are trained first. They may receive this training at workshops, seminars, or facilities that have ongoing, active programs. Visiting consultants represent a viable alternative. Experienced trainers or educators may not need this outside help. For them, review of the literature may suffice.

Leaders can be trained by the facilitators or outside experts; but it is important that the other members get their training from the circle leader.[1] The leader's first task is to allay fears and persuade his or her teammates to volunteer.

THE QC MEETING

An Agenda for Members

1. History, concept, and benefits of QCs
2. Description of proposed program
3. Team development
4. Basic meeting skills
5. Problem-solving techniques
6. Communication skills
7. Planning skills

Additional Agenda for Leaders

1. Why some managers fear QCs
2. How QCs benefit managers and employees
3. Participative leadership styles
4. Planning, leading and evaluating a QC meeting
5. Pitfalls
6. How to teach members

Time and Place for Meetings

The meetings should take place at least monthly. Less often is usually unwise. It may be difficult to find a suitable meeting site and get the members together. Therefore, the selection of the right day, time, and place is very important. Pick days when the work load is lightest. If members are from different shifts, the best time may be late in the afternoon when the shifts change.

The usual allotted time is 1 hour. While this may be modified, major variation from meeting to meeting should not be great. After an hour, people grow restless. Their minds turn to other responsibilities. Leaders must be sensitive to the wishes and schedules of the members.

Routine Problem Solving

1. Determine if the problem merits study by asking these questions:
   Does it affect many people or many laboratory results?
   Is there a significant safety risk?
   If uncorrected, may legal action follow?
   Is there a large monetary factor?
   Is a special client or client group affected?
   What is the potential for correction?
   Can this circle handle it?
2. Analyze the problem:
   collect and collate data.
   review literature on subject.
   review historical handling of problem.
   have individual members study collated data.
   have group study data.

   Ideally, much of the data come from customers. The sources and methodology of these collections were discussed in Chapter 1. The techniques of problem solving, including the use of cause-and-effect diagrams, Pareto charts, and "brainstorming," will be discussed in Chapter 6.
3. Develop alternative solutions, and pick the best one.
4. Make a presentation or send a report to management.
5. Review action by management.
6. Follow up.

MEASURING RESULTS

The QC must have a solid baseline against which to measure results. Data that represent outcome are best. Examples are degrees of accuracy or precision, turnaround time, and number of documented customer complaints. Data that represent behavior or process rather than outcome or results are less solid. Ratings of turnover, attendance, and performance may reflect attitudes and job satisfaction, but statistical validity is difficult to achieve.

IMPLEMENTATION, REPORTS, AND FOLLOW-UP

Start with a pilot program. Select a laboratory unit that has historically demonstrated its flexibility and adaptability. Begin with a relatively simple problem: one with a high potential for success that is highly visible and provides the group with a feeling of accomplishment.

Reports can be submitted by the facilitator, the leader, or a recorder. The reports should include recommendations and alternative solutions. Specific data such as estimated cost, a timetable, and personnel involved should be included, as well as notes of potential barriers.

Presentations may be made to management by the circle leader, or by the entire group. The latter is better because it gives each member the opportunity to present a specific part of the report.[1]

Subsequent administrative actions and results are discussed and recorded. Each project merits a separate report, including follow-up data. The monitoring process may continue indefinitely, or may be finalized, in which case the report is transferred to an inactive file.

PITFALLS

Many QCs fail. That is not surprising when one considers the many pitfalls. Here is a list of some of these pitfalls (the asterisks indicate the most common ones). Please note that most represent managerial deficiencies:

Lack of top management commitment and support
Employee or supervisor resistance to change
Failure to obtain employee commitment
Inadequate training
Understaffing*
Failure to use trained facilitators
Poor leadership. Meetings can easily degenerate into gripe sessions
Lack of incentives
Scheduling problems*
Union resistance or animosity of employees toward management
Poor communication
Inadequate meeting area or frequent interruptions*
Selection of inappropriate topics
Impractical recommendations
One or more members dominate or sabotage meetings
Lack of action on recommendations

REFERENCES

1. Thompson PC: *Quality Circles: How to Make Them Work in America.* New York, AMACOM, Book Division, 1982.
2. Lawler EE, Mohrman SA: Quality circles after the fad. *Harvard Bus Rev* 1985;63:64–71.
3. Ross MB, Hass B: Applying Japanese management styles in American hospitals: Focus on values. *Hosp Prog* 1984;64:45–49.
4. Waszak JJ: Adapting QCs to health care: Some special challenges. *Hosp Prog* 1982;63:47.

5. Helmer FT, Gunatilake S: A supervisor's tool for solving operational problems in nursing. *Health Care Super* 1988;6:63–71.

6. Jimenez JF, Turley CP, Quiggins CS: A quality circle improves pediatric phlebotomy. *MLO* 1988;20:85–87.

7. Wellstood SA, Wright L: Using quality circles to spot and solve lab problems. *MLO* 1983;15:32–40.

8. Orbaugh PK, Orbaugh K: Is your lab ready for quality circles? *MLO* 1983;15:41–48.

9. Diamond I: Quality circles in the clinical laboratory. *Pathologist* 1984;6:95–98.

10. Tilley K: Putting quality circles to work in chemistry. *MLO* 1987;19:41–49.

11. Sims HP Jr, Dean JW Jr: Beyond quality circles: Self-managing teams. *Personnel* 1985;62:25–41.

12. Schwabbauer M, CE Work Group, Dept of Pathology, University of Iowa: A useful strategy. *MLO* 1990;22:54–60.

13. Roethlisberger F, Dickson W: *Management and the Worker.* Cambridge, Mass, Harvard University Press, 1939.

6. Problem Solving

THE RATE AND complexity of technological, legal, organizational and regulatory changes is increasing. Customer expectations and litigiousness have increased. Personnel shortages and fiscal restraints have burgeoned and require creative decision making. Successful EPGs such as quality circles demand it.

DECISION MAKING AND GROUP PROBLEM SOLVING

Judgment involves analytical thinking, logic, intuition, and creativity. Without intuition we would not have much that is worthy of analysis. Without analytical powers our imaginations would leap to wild and reckless conclusions. [1]

Do not underestimate the value of a third element, experience. It is the only source of true vision. Intuition is largely experience stored in our subconscious minds. Group problem solving capitalizes on the combined experience of all of the group's members.

There are two major advantages to group problem solving. First, by synergism more ideas are generated. Second, when members of a group select solutions, they are more likely to support that choice.

People support what they help to create.

THE CHARGE TO A PROBLEM-SOLVING GROUP

The convening authority states not only what is to be achieved, but also what must be avoided, eg, "We want to decrease the turnaround time without sacrificing quality, or purchasing new equipment."[1] (The quality circle usually selects its own subject matter.)

Preliminary Questions

Are the topics selected by the convening authority, the group leader, or the group?
Is the group to submit a list of alternative solutions, or only the solution it chooses?
Is there a target date for a report?
What facilities and budget for expenses are available?
Will the group's recommendations be implemented, or are they for information only?

The last question is especially important if the cooperation of the group is to be maintained. What is articulated can be critical. For example, if the manager says "We must come up with a decision at this meeting," the group will think that its decision will be implemented. If it is not, then the group's enthusiasm at future problem-solving meetings will be nil. The manager should have said "I need your input to pass on to the higher authorities."

THE NINE KEY STEPS TO PROBLEM SOLVING

1. Prepare a Problem Statement

Jumping to conclusions leads to unhappy landings.

Managers often shortchange this step in their haste to arrive at a solution.

Key Questions

Is this situation really a problem?
Is this a problem or only the symptom of a bigger problem?
Does it require our attention?
Is it a minor problem that can be corrected without a comprehensive analysis?

A problem well stated is a problem partly solved.

2. Get and Interpret the Facts

The quality of decisions is directly proportional to the number of relevant facts. Judgment is required to determine when sufficient information has been acquired. People with scientific backgrounds tend to procrastinate because they want all of the data that are available. They fall prey to the "jigsaw puzzle fallacy"; *ie*, there is only one correct decision (the puzzle must have four straight edges). But management decisions tend to be gray rather than black or white, and often there are several good solutions.

Address the who, where, when, what, why, and how of the situation by asking questions.

When was the problem first observed?
What are its manifestations?
Who is affected or involved?
Where is this taking place?
Is it getting better or worse?
What is the real cause? To get at that, ask a series of "Whys?"

3. State Your Objectives

What would the ideal solution be?
Absolute requirement: What is the least satisfactory solution that is acceptable?

4. Generate Alternatives

The greater the number of alternatives considered, the greater the chance that one will be satisfactory. It is during this step that creative solutions should supplement logic and experience.

Do not overlook any alternative, even if it appears unattractive at first blush. Also, remember that one choice that is always available is to do nothing.

Example: The nursing staff complains that fasting blood sugar reports are late. You have performed step 2, gathering the necessary information, determining when specimen collections start, the number of phlebotomists, when specimens arrive in the laboratory, when processing starts, when results are available, and how the results are transmitted to the nursing stations.

Here are some alternative solutions to be considered:

Ignore the complaints. The service compares favorably with that of competitors.
Ask physicians to delay the time of their rounds (humor!).
Begin collecting earlier.
Beef up the phlebotomy team.
Assign fewer patients to novice collectors.
Purchase a faster glucose analyzer.
Telephone reports.
Request nursing personnel to send messengers to pick up reports in the laboratory.
Recommend a data processing system.

5. Formulate Criteria to Evaluate the Alternatives

Absolute Criteria

These usually begin with "must," eg, "must be put into effect by . . ." or "maximum cost must be less than . . .".

Differential Criteria

Additional criteria are needed to compare those alternatives that meet the absolute prerequisites. These criteria may relate to cost, convenience, or acceptance. They can be given weighted numbers, eg: turnaround time, 5; patients' comfort, 5; and least change in work patterns, 2.

6. Evaluate the Alternatives

Compare each alternative with the criteria established in the previous step. Do not overlook the possibility of combining solutions.

7. Troubleshoot the Selection

Ask what could go wrong. Use a lot of "what ifs." Devil's advocates or conscientious worriers are valuable at this point. They keep the group from venturing into fantasyland, and ensure thorough consideration of the risks involved.[1]

8. Develop an Action Plan

Include in your plan sequenced action steps, a time schedule, a list of needed resources, and specific assignments for employees who will implement the plan.
  Ask these three questions[1]:

1. Have all alternatives been considered?
2. Have all possible consequences of each alternative been considered?
3. Have contingencies been provided for?

(**A caveat:** Do not discard all the paperwork. If the recommended solution falters, it may be necessary to go back and start all over again.)

9. The Follow-Up

Architects have not discharged their responsibilities when their blueprints have been submitted. Plans must be interpreted, progress inspected, and variances noted. The same is true of problem solvers. Check to see if the solution is producing the desired results. Do not be afraid to admit to mistakes. Chalk them up to experience.

THE "SALAMI" APPROACH TO COMPLEX PROBLEMS

Sometimes a problem seems overwhelming and the group becomes confused and frustrated. When this ensues, pick out one relatively simple part of the problem and lead the group to a solution. Later, as larger slices are taken, the problem will appear less threatening.

THREE PROBLEM-SOLVING TRAPS

1. The statement of the problem is too restrictive. This leads to the exclusion of some alternatives.
   Example:
   "Should we recommend a backup instrument?" (poor)
   "What's the best way to handle instrument downtime?" (better)
2. Biases. A previous experience affects the present decision.
3. The confirmation trap. When a tentative decision is made, there is a tendency to look only for evidence that confirms that decision, ignoring evidence that may challenge that decision.

USEFUL TOOLS IN PROBLEM SOLVING

SWOT analysis is a useful tool for analyzing special situations, problems or threats. It is particularly helpful when studying a new service, or modifying an existing one. The situation is scrutinized from four aspects:

Strengths of the organization and its personnel
Weaknesses of the organization and its personnel
Opportunities provided by the situation
Threats from competition or opponents

Cost/benefit analysis is the ratio of the cost of an alternative to its benefit or profit. For example: in comparing two instruments, it has been determined that instrument A costs $50,000 and its use would yield an annual profit of $100,000. Instrument B costs $35,000 and would generate a profit of $75,000.

Cost/benefit ratio of instrument A:
   50,000/100,000 = 0.50
Cost/benefit ratio of instrument B:
   35,000/75,000 = 0.47 (better)

Once a problem has been clearly enunciated, major causal categories can be depicted in a cause and effect ("fishbone") diagram. These categories are broken down and listed on the chart, as shown in Figure 6.1.[2] The problem is then addressed by focusing on one category at a time.

Pareto charts are useful in depicting the relative importance of various factors (Figure 6.2).[2]

Laboratorians are familiar with flow charts such as the one shown in Figure 6.3.[3] The Gantt chart is a graph with activities listed on the vertical axis, and time units listed on the horizontal axis (Figure 6.4).[3]

Histograms, scatter diagrams, and Deming control charts are also useful.

GROUP BRAINSTORMING

The main features of brainstorming are cross stimulation, suspended judgment, and the special setting.[4] Cross stimulation is achieved because the members have different perspectives.

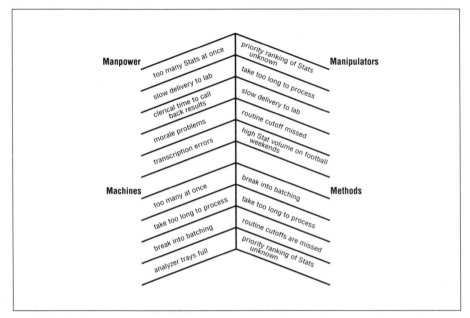

Figure 6.1 A cause-and-effect (fishbone) diagram. (Reprinted, by permission, from Tilley KL: Putting quality circles to work in chemistry. *MLO* 1987;19:42–49.)

In well-directed brainstorming sessions, judgment of ideas is prohibited during the idea-generation phase. The following types of attempts are spiked by the leader or facilitator:

"That won't work because . . ."
"You can't be serious."
"We could never get that approved."
"That's too risky."

The special setting of the meeting provides an opportunity for people to make suggestions that they would otherwise not dare to make for fear of being laughed at. In a brainstorming session, anything goes.[4]

The Technique of Group Brainstorming

The Generation Phase

Get off to a good start by describing the topic before the meeting. Set a good example by bringing a large packet of ideas, including some wild ones. This encourages others to do likewise.

Each member writes down all his or her suggestions on a sheet of paper. Call on each person for one suggestion. Go around the table until all ideas are offered. Write down the ideas on a flip chart as they are offered.

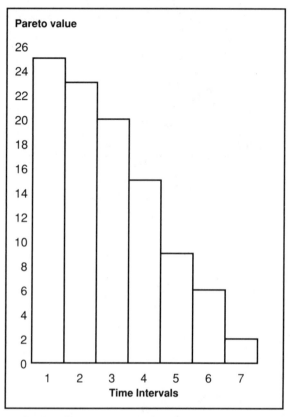

Pareto analysis of Stats

Busiest Stat time Intervals	% of tests that are Stat electrolytes	Pareto value
1. 3 a.m.– 5 a.m.	99	25
2. 5 a.m.– 8 a.m.	91	23
3. 7 p.m.– 3 a.m.	80	20
4. 5 p.m.– 7 p.m.	60	15
5. 12 p.m.– 5 p.m.	35	9
6. 11 a.m.–12 p.m.	23	6
7. 8 a.m.–11 a.m.	10	2
	Total: 398	

Pareto value = Frequency of an item (expressed as %) + total

Figure 6.2 Pareto chart. (Reprinted, by permission, from Tilley KL: Putting quality circles to work in chemistry. *MLO* 1987;19:42–49.)

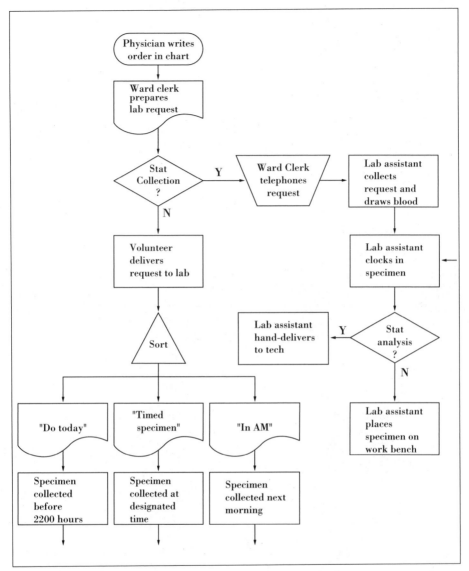

Figure 6.3 Flowchart for blood specimen collection. (Reprinted, by permission, from Umiker WO: *The Effective Laboratory Supervisor*. Oradell, NJ, Medical Economics Co, 1982.)

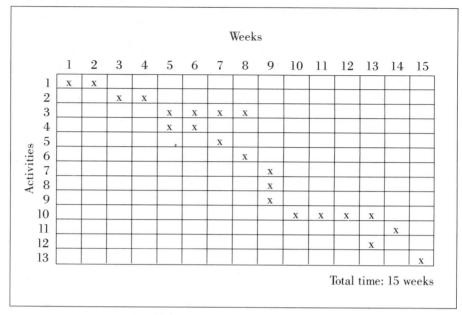

Figure 6.4 Gantt chart. (Reproduced, by permission, from Umiker WO: *The Effective Laboratory Supervisor.* Oradell, NJ, Medical Economics Co, 1982.)

No judgments are made, positive or negative, but members may "piggyback" suggestions onto those of other members. Participants are encouraged to add to their lists as the suggestions of others are being offered.

The Evaluation Phase

Creativity now gives way to judgment. The pros and cons are discussed. Start with the positives. For instance, ask "What's good about this idea?" If you do not come up with anything positive, go on to the next one.

Do not discuss the negatives until all of the positives have been expressed. Do not defend your own ideas (at least at first). Let the others carry the ball. If the idea is good, you will not be the only one who recognizes it.

Criticism should be phrased in a positive way. Here is a good way to express doubt about a suggestion without discouraging the person: instead of saying "no," or "yes, but," try the IPC technique of Glassman[5]:

Interest: express some in the idea.
Positive: focus on a positive aspect of the idea.
Concerns: state yours instead of stating disapproval. Example: "Sue, I'm concerned about how your proposal may affect the night shift."

When someone responds: "we tried that and it didn't work," answer with "what's different this time?" or "how can those obstacles be overcome?"

SEEKING A CONSENSUS

Strive for unanimity, settle for consensus and avoid voting.

A group often makes decisions before all the opinions of the members have been explored. Outranked, outvoted, or unheard-from participants may leave angry, balk at the decision, fail to support it, or even sabotage its implementation.

A consensus is a genuine meeting of the minds. It is not reached by voting. Some members may prefer solutions other than the one decided upon, but they concede that they had ample time to express their feelings, and that the decision was arrived at after full and fair discussion. They feel that they can live with the selected alternative.

Three Strong Features of Consensus Reaching

1. Full participation by all members.
2. Avoidance of hasty decisions.
3. Gaining the support of participants in implementing the decision.

Rules of Consensus Decision Making

1. Everyone voices his or her view completely.
2. The positive features of each alternative are emphasized.
3. Hasty agreements are avoided.
4. Negative features are exposed and analyzed.
5. Disagreements are resolved.
6. Voting is avoided.
7. Each member agrees that he or she can support the solution that is accepted.
   Finally, each participant privately ranks the suggestions numerically, and the rankings are added up.

REFERENCES

1. Heirs B, Farrell P: *Professional Decision Thinker*. New York, Dodd Mead & Co, 1986.
2. Tilley KL: Putting quality circles to work in chemistry. *MLO* 1987;19:41–49.
3. Umiker WO: *The Effective Laboratory Supervisor*. Oradell, NJ, Medical Economics Co, 1982.
4. DeBono E: *Lateral Thinking: Creativity Step-by-Step*. New York, Harper & Row, 1970.
5. Glassman E: Creative problem solving: Your role as leader. *Supervis Manage* 34:4 April 1989;34:37–42.

7. Position Descriptions and Performance Standards

PROFESSIONAL ATHLETES DO not have written position descriptions, but they know precisely what they must do, and how well to do it. Institutions use position descriptions and work standards to spell out these two essentials for their employees.

Often performance is unsatisfactory because employees simply do not know what they are supposed to do. How can we expect good performance when we hand newly hired persons outdated position descriptions, rush them through a shoddy indoctrination program, and then tell them: "If you don't hear from me, you're doing just fine." In this chapter we will introduce customer service items into position descriptions and performance standards.

THE POSITION SUMMARY

The position summary, also called the "umbrella statement," "position purpose," and "function statement," is a segment of the job description that condenses the responsibilities of the incumbent. It may include the goal, reporting channel, and other job features. For example:

"Plans, directs and controls a ten-person hematology section of a clinical laboratory. Responsible also for the teaching of students and new employees. Performs wide range of diagnostic hematologic procedures. Reports to a laboratory manager."

Insert the word "customer" somewhere in the summary statement. In the above example, you might add, "The major goal of this position is to meet or exceed customer expectations. Customers include patients, patient's families and visitors, clinicians and other care providers, third-party payers, teammates, students and trainees, and hospital departments or committees served by the laboratory."

QUALIFICATIONS

Qualifications describe the requirements of the job, not the qualifications of the job holder. This includes the abilities and traits that the incumbent must have, and what you *hope* he or she has.

For some jobs, the major qualifications can be abbreviated because they are spelled out in the mandatory education, training, and registration, or licensure requirements of that specialty, eg, "registered MT (ASCP) or equivalent."

Special prerequisites are stated. For example, a medical transcriptionist must be familiar with medical terminology. Other specifications are less susceptible to validation. Temperament, traits, and personality are important but highly subjective. Justification of their inclusion must be provided in the subsequent descriptions of duties and responsibilities.

Smart[1] claims that for most technical or staff positions at least 15 personal specifications are required. These include characteristics such as learning ability, analysis skills, judgment, honesty, loyalty, emotional stability, maturity, friendliness, and so forth.

Special Demands

In the client-oriented laboratory, we go beyond technical skills and delineate the personal traits we seek. Delineate areas of special importance or sensitivity. Articulate the major items in behavioral terms. For example:

"Is discrete with patient information."
"Shows composure under stress."
"Demonstrates accuracy in reporting results."
"Accepts night and weekend assignments."
"Exhibits skill and proficiency in applying technical principles and techniques relating to medical technology."
"Recognizes lab safety risks and minimizes danger to self and to coworkers."

This is a golden opportunity to inject customer awareness. Add specifications such as "recognizes or anticipates needs of customers," and "comprehends and practices the principles of guest relations."

PEOPLE RELATIONSHIPS

The reporting relationship identifies an incumbent's immediate superior, and other managers to whom he or she is directly accountable.

Special departmental and interdepartmental relationships coordinate the operational aspects. For example, a blood bank supervisor must have special concern for the emergency room and the surgical suite. He or she must coordinate tasks with laboratory sections such as hematology and serology. For example:

"Peer relationships with other laboratory supervisors, office manager and quality assurance coordinator."
"Advises technical director of school."
"Consults with director of hospital information systems."

Customer relationships are, for the most part, delineated in other segments of the position description. However, some key statements may be appropriately stated here. For example:

"Maintains confidentiality of medical and personal information."
"Serves as resource person and role model."
"Participates in committees, quality circles, and other problem-solving groups."
"Reports customer complaints to superiors."
"Anticipates operational problems and responds promptly and effectively."
"Shares knowledge and expertise willingly."

RESPONSIBILITIES, DUTIES, AND TASKS

Each responsibility should be accompanied by a statement that describes the type of behavior or outcome that identifies successful job performance. These descriptors serve as performance criteria. Content validity is established because these criteria are based on observable work behaviors or results rather than traits.

List responsibilities in order of importance, or the percentage of time needed. Responsibilities describe activities in their broadest sense, while tasks describe them in the most specific terms. For example:

Responsibility: "Teach MLT students"
Duty: "Provide benchwork instruction for twenty 3-hour sessions"
Tasks: "Prepare agenda, demonstrate method, grade students"

Subdivision of duties makes more work and lengthens documents. However, the effort is often worthwhile when the position description is of a job in which detailed instructions are helpful, eg, one filled by an individual who has limited cognitive skills, or no previous experience.

Select the most descriptive terminology, using action verbs when possible. Take into account (1) clarification of the duty, (2) the self-esteem of the employee, and (3) the effect of the terminology on the salary classification. Consider the following alternatives:

"Makes visitors feel welcome" for "greet people."[2]
"Evaluates laboratory results" for "checks laboratory results."
"Establishes comprehensive quality controls that prevent release of erroneous information" for "sets quality controls."

Useful Verbs for Position Descriptions

Apply (current knowledge)
Arrange (meeting room)

Calibrate (instruments)
Design (new work flow)
Determine (suitable methods)
Establish (procedures for)
Evaluate (usefulness of new instruments)
Instruct (orientees)
Maintain (systems for documenting)
Monitor (work of new employees)
Perform (tests)
Process (specimens)
Promote (public relations)
Recognize (errors)
Record (statistical results)
Report (violations)
Select (new employees)

PERFORMANCE STANDARDS

When you have updated the basic position description, you are ready to formulate the performance standards. Performance standards have two cardinal uses. The first is to inform employees *how well* they must do their work, since the basic job description states only *what* is expected, and the necessary qualifications. The second use is to facilitate performance evaluations, especially if a pay-for-performance strategy is in place. Without performance standards, employee evaluations are highly subjective, and this can lead to charges of discrimination.

All employees have the following questions about their responsibilities, whether or not they articulate them:

"Exactly what do you want me to do?"
"How well and how fast must I do these things?"
"How can I learn new skills?"
"How am I doing?"

Position descriptions and performance standards address the first two of these queries directly, and lay the foundation for responding to the other two.

Performance Levels

Some organizations use three levels. Standards for these systems are easiest to administer. These three levels are:

1. Does not meet expectations (fails).
2. Meets expectations (passes).
3. Exceeds expectations (excels).

For certain behavioral factors, there can only be two levels, satisfactory and unsatisfactory. For example, an employee does or does not steal, use drugs, or reveal confidential information.

In the five-tiered system, one of the additional categories is "meets expecta-tions, but needs improvement" (or, "below average"). The fifth class is derived by splitting the "exceeds expectations" group into "superior" (or "above average") and "outstanding." Anyone who has been faced with an indignant overachiever who wants to know why he or she is rated as "superior" instead of "outstanding" appreciates the difficulty of using a five-level system.

Importance of Setting Appropriate Levels

A minimum-level standard provides a fail-pass situation. Performance below that level is unacceptable, signaling a need for remedial or administrative action. If this level is too low, it leads to the acceptance of poor performance and the accumulation of "deadwood."

On the other hand, if the level is too high there may be frustration and loss of self-esteem when standards are not met. According to one writer, when there is an 80% chance of meeting a performance standard, that standard has a challenging effect. When that percentage drops to 50% or less, the standard becomes incapacitating.[3]

The Three Kinds of Standards

Compliance Standards

Compliance standards concern employee obedience to policies and procedures. They relate to attendance, punctuality, appearance, and so forth.

Compliance standards need not be duplicated in position descriptions. Dispose of them with a global statement like "complies with the conditions of employment described in the Personnel Policy and Procedures Manual."[4]

While you need not duplicate these criteria, variations from what is pre-scribed in personnel manuals may be necessary. For example, the dress code for phlebotomists may be more stringent than that for employees who have no patient contact.

Temperament and Interrelationship Standards

Work habits, initiative, creativity, self-development, reliability, and communica-tion skills are governed by temperament and interrelationship standards. These standards rely on "soft data" because they are highly subjective. Most of them cannot be tied directly to specific tasks, and therefore are posited in a special segment of the position description.

Although these standards for behavior and traits are often omitted from position descriptions, they invariably show up in performance evaluation forms, much to the embarassment of the raters.

Task Standards

Task standards are based on outcome and results. They utilize "hard data," since most of them are objective. Examples are turnaround time, infection rates, and compliance with budget. There are five dimensions of task standards:

1. quality (errors, precision, accuracy)
2. quantity (productivity rate, tests per day)
3. timeliness (deadlines, turnaround time)
4. cost effectiveness (budget, cost per test)
5. manner of performance (courtesy, cooperation)

The simplest means of formulating a task standard is to list the major duties, then add appropriate descriptors that represent one or more of the five dimensions. For example:

Task: Answer telephone
Standards:
1. Provides complete information sought by callers. Ensures that transfer calls are completed. (Quality)
2. Keeps lines open by processing calls expeditiously and avoiding personal calls. (Quantity)
3. Answers calls within three rings. (Timeliness)
4. Identifies department and self. Asks "how can I help?" Uses caller's name frequently. Closes by thanking caller. (Manner of performance)

Do not be discouraged when classification of descriptors is not as precise as you would like, as long as the information appears in the document. Periodic modifications dictated by experience are a key to success.[5]

Quantify When Possible

The introduction of numbers and percentages adds to objectivity. More importantly, accuracy of description is increased. "Answer within three rings" is very precise, "answer promptly" is not. Percentages indicate the amount of tolerance or the number of errors that is permitted. This can be important. Consider "answer within three rings" and "correctly crossmatch blood." "Ninety percent of the time" would be appropriate for the number of telephone rings allowed, but is intolerable for accuracy of compatibility testing.

Often it is not possible or advantageous to apply percentages. In fact, objections to their use have been voiced on the grounds that one would have to record each episode before percentages could be calculated. That would convert every supervisor into a "bean counter."

There is no interpretive problem with terms like "always," "never" or "without exception." But there is a problem of achievement. Even our best employees slip once in a while. Therefore terms like "with rare exception" are preferable to absolute terms.[4]

The adverbs "generally," "ordinarily," or "usually" equate to over 50%, while "sometimes," "seldom," or "infrequently" denote occurrences below 50%.[5]

Focus on Quality Assurance and Consumer Factors by Using Word Searches

Below is a list of terms that identify a quality assurance statement, followed by a list that pertains to customer satisfaction. If your position descriptions are stored on word processors, word searches can be accomplished quickly, and if the following words are sparse, your position descriptions probably should be upgraded.

Quality assurance words

precision	accuracy	statistic
error	downtime	budget
overtime	cost	abnormal
proficiency	expense	forecast
analyze	mistake	inspect
calculate	monitor	collate
measure	tabulate	verify
troubleshoot	sign out	range
variance	outlier	normal

Customer-oriented words

participate	negotiate	coordinate
correlate	guide	inform
interpret	interview	train
sooth	volunteer	satisfy
comfort	complaints	indoctrinate
grievance	support	communicate
morale	encourage	reassure
assist	commend	criticize
listen	please	anger

Some General Customer-Oriented Performance Standards

Is tactful in personal interactions.
Communicates in honest, straightforward manner.
Reports employee concerns to lab management.
Reacts constructively to criticism and to changes.
Maintains high team spirit and morale.
Interacts positively.
Rarely complained about by clients or staff.
Client information is always kept confidential.

Some Specific Customer-Oriented Performance Standards

Phlebotomist

With rare exception[6]:

appearance, dress and decorum conform to special laboratory code.
greets patients courteously by introducing self and calling patient by name.
explains procedure about to be performed.
complies with institutional policies and procedures with special attention to isolation procedures.

Microbiology Technologist

With rare exception[6]:

corrects errors before reports leave laboratory.
maintains good rapport and cooperative working relationship with members of the other laboratory sections.
demonstrates enthusiasm even when complex time-consuming tests are ordered on days when section is short-staffed.

Blood Bank Technician

With rare exception:

maintains good rapport with other laboratory employees. Knows them all by name.[6]
handles telephone requests expeditiously and courteously even during stressful situations.
maintains good working relationships with members of the emergency room, critical care units, and surgical suite.

REFERENCES

1. Smart BD: *The Smart Interviewer: Tools and Techniques for Hiring the Best.* New York, John Wiley & Sons, 1989.
2. Cathcart J: Winning customer service. *Management Sol* 1988:33;10–17.
3. Hochheiser RM: *How to Work for a Jerk.* New York, Vantage Publishers, 1987.
4. Berte L: *Developing Performance Standards for Hospital Personnel.* Chicago, ASCP Press, 1989.
5. Umiker W, Yohe S: *Performance Standards for Laboratory Personnel.* Oradell, NJ, Medical Economics Co, 1984.
6. *The Criteria Based Job Description and Performance Evaluation System.* Wheeling, Ill, Personal and Professional Development Inc, 1985.

8. Selecting Customer-Oriented Personnel

I**T'S A LOT** easier to hire the right people to begin with than to try to fix them later.[1] Institutions that lead in customer service take pains to hire people whose personalities predispose them to serve clients well. Professional recruiters use interviews, hypothetical situations, and psychological tests to screen applicants.[2] Our goal is to hire people who have demonstrated the right customer service attitude in their previous work and social conduct. This is based on the assumption that past performance is the best indicator of future comportment. Once a person has been hired, it is much easier to reinforce good attitudes than it is to change bad ones.

To get the kind of employees we want, there are three imperatives. First, there must be an effective recruiting program. We want a lot of good candidates. Second, the selection process should enable us to pick the best candidate with a high degree of confidence. Third, we must succeed in getting the candidates of our choice to accept our offers.

First-line supervisors have little influence on the recruiting practices of their organizations, but they play a major role in the interviewing process, and in persuading candidates to join their teams.

RECRUITMENT MODALITIES

Cast a very wide net and carefully sift through what you catch in it.[3]

Employees who are self-recruited or are recommended by current employees, or who have served as volunteers or student interns, have a higher retention rate and perform better than those who are obtained through other modalities.

Recruitment materials should be prepared by professionals, since a poorly handled brochure can be so inadequate that it actually turns off prospective candidates.[4]

INSTRUMENTS FOR EVALUATING CANDIDATES

Application forms and resumes are of limited value. Special questionnaires that are tailored specifically to certain positions are more informative.[5]

Resumes are candidates' public relations sheets, ie, balance sheets without liabilities. When studying resumes, look for items that reflect customer service, such as successful sales jobs, volunteer work, participation in team athletics, active membership in social organizations, and responsibilities that exceed job requirements. Verification of credentials is a given. There must be confirmation of licensure, certification, or registration.

"Some of the best fiction writing in the world is in the form of resumes."[6]

Preemployment tests can be helpful, but are underutilized. Employers do not like to take the time to administer these, or they may be afraid of violating antidiscrimination laws, knowing that managers must be able to prove that the tests possess validity and reliability. As long as a test is based on a required skill or knowledge as documented in the job description, such fears are groundless. For example:

A phlebotomist candidate may be asked to role play in a blood collection procedure.

A clerk-receptionist candidate takes some incoming phone calls.

A laboratory technician candidate who will have teaching responsibilities is forewarned that all candidates must give a short lecture or bench work demonstration.

Special questionnaires that are purported to measure honesty, loyalty, and positive attitudes are now available, but the jury is still out on their usefulness.

QUESTIONS AND MORE QUESTIONS

Interviewers tend to ask more questions that deal with technical skill and experience rather than with people skills. While this may well be an error by employers generally, it is a "fatal flaw" for those trying to develop a customer-oriented laboratory. Every interview question can be used to evaluate crucial people skills.

Kinds of Questions

1. Close-ended questions are those that can be answered in one or a few words, eg, "When are you available?" These questions are used to get basic data,

but should not be used to elicit detailed information. You will not learn much from a question such as "Did you like your last supervisor?"

2. Open-ended questions cannot be answered with a few words, and are much better for obtaining detailed information. Change the above closed-ended question to "Tell me about your last supervisor" and you will learn a lot more.

3. Introductory questions start information flowing. For example: "Tell me about a work crisis you faced." (Not: "Can you handle a crisis?") This is an introductory, open-ended question.

4. Probing questions address the five Ws: why, what, who, when, and where. These are excellent, but if overused create a dialogue that sounds like a grilling. For example: "How did that situation arise?" "Why was that allowed to happen? How did your supervisor respond? In retrospect, what would you have done differently?" (Probing questions that build on the introductory question)

5. Hypothetical questions, eg, "What would you do if . . .". These situational queries can be very informative.

6. Illegal questions must be avoided. They are prohibited by federal and state statutes. If you do not have a list of these, get one from your human resources department before you interview the next candidate.

7. Knockout questions address items that automatically eliminate candidates, eg, for lack of licensure or unwillingness to work weekends.[7]

8. Questions related to general duties. Use the position description and job specifications (qualifications) to formulate questions regarding education, training, experience, knowledge, and skill. There are some excellent books on this subject.[1,7,8]

9. Questions to evaluate general service attitudes and behavior. The examples given below reflect a broad spectrum of traits and qualities including judgment, maturity, emotional stability, teamwork, and flexibility.

"Tell me about your school attendance record. Did you have trouble getting to 8-AM classes? On the average, how many school days did you miss each year?" (For a recent graduate)

"How often were you late for work?" "Describe your attendance record." (Candidate had previous jobs)

"When did you have trouble meeting deadlines?" "How often was that?"

"What would you do about reporting a 'panic value' when you can't reach the attending physician?"

"Describe your participation in team sports and social activities at school."

"How would you describe your 'followership' style?"

"Give me an example of how you adjusted to change."

"What work situations at your last job required special patience and tact?"

"How do you feel about overtime? Call-backs? Extra-hour assignments?"

"What are some risks you took at work during the past year?"

"Give me a couple of examples of your creativity."

"What is the best and the worst decision you made recently?"

10. Questions to specifically evaluate interpersonal skills and customer service attitude. Picture the ideal candidates. What are they doing? What are they saying to clients? What is their body language like? How do they react to coworkers? Use these images to formulate appropriate questions.

"What do you do when a nurse becomes insulting on the telephone?"

"Give me an example of how you made an extra effort to please a client."

"How do you think a laboratory can provide better patient service?"

"How do you think a laboratory can improve its relationship with the nursing service?"

"How would you go about finding out how customers feel about laboratory service?"

"Did you ever take care of a chronically ill relative? Tell me about it."

"Did you ever work in a nursing home? Tell me about it."

"How would your boss and your fellow workers rate your teamwork (friendliness, cooperation)? Why?"

"Describe your participation in community committee activities."

"What kind of people or things irritate you? How did you handle them?"

"Give me an example of how you dealt with severe or unjust criticism."

"Describe a situation in which your integrity was challenged."

"Are you assertive? Tell me about a situation in which you were assertive."

"How would you describe your participation at a meeting?"

"How many times have you lost your cool in the past month? Tell me about one of these."

"Give me an example of how you demonstrated a 'caring attitude.'"

THE INTERVIEW

Preparation Checklist

1. Familiarize yourself with the position description. Concentrate on the duties and required qualifications.
2. Review the application and resume.
3. Prepare the list of questions you are going to ask and review those interdicted by law.
4. Prepare a list of positive features of the job. Know the salary and benefits.
5. Visualize the tour of your facilities that you will provide, and alert the people whom you want the candidate to meet.
6. Schedule a time and place with privacy and freedom from interruptions.

First Impressions

Your first impression of a job applicant is also how the customer will see him or her.[3]

Handling Sensitive Issues

Be tactful when you probe the soft spots. Start by stating that one of the ways you evaluate maturity is by the ability of people to recognize and talk about performance areas that could be improved. Point out that such people have already taken the first step toward career improvement.

Avoid strong words like "weakness," "deficiency," and "shortcoming." Substitute words like "area of concern," "need for more experience," or "enhance full potential." Use softeners such as "might, perhaps, and somewhat" and phrases such as "is it possible that . . .? How did you happen to . . .?" For example (a little overdone): "Could it be, Pat, that at times, you're inclined to delay a bit?"

Comments About Evaluation of Candidates

Assume people will change only if they have demonstrated this ability in the past.
Weigh negatives more heavily than positives. A lack of negatives is one of the most important factors in success.
Watch for strong feelings and beliefs. They indicate rigidity and intolerance.
Note where the candidate's emphasis is. Customer-oriented people talk about service and interpersonal relationships. Task-oriented individuals focus on duties. Burned-out workaholics use the word "stress" frequently.
Do not leap to conclusions.

How to Recognize the Untruthful Ones

1. Their resumes and comments seem too good to be true. They appear to be overqualified for the job.
2. Their employment record fails to show real progression.
3. They gloss over deficiencies and exaggerate almost every competency.
4. Their body language gives them away.
5. They give poor responses to challenging questions related to qualifications.

Closing the Interview

Ask for the person's level of interest, eg, "While neither of us is in a position to make a decision at this point, what's your level of interest?" (good) "Are you interested in the job?" (not as good)

Explore doubts or reservations. If the person is noncommittal and is a good candidate, set a deadline for his or her answer.

Tell the candidate when the selection decision will be made, who will make it, and how the notification will be done. Make certain that you have the person's current telephone number and address.

Take candidates to their next interview, other on-site destination, or the exit closest to their transportation. Thank them for coming.

Record your observations immediately after the meeting and before another interview. Make note of any information that seems to be lacking.

How to Maximize Your Chances of Signing on the Candidate

Remember that the better the candidate, the more competition for his or her services. To be in the running, you must be enthusiastic and persuasive, yet be perceived as honest and sincere.

1. Send a map and directions for getting to the interview site. State what, if any, reimbursement for travel is provided. This demonstrates a caring attitude. It also gets your interview off to a good start.
2. Establish the right ambience.
   It gets you more and better data.
   It elicits a smoother dialogue.
   It increases the acceptance rate by candidates.
   It creates goodwill toward the organization.
   Candidates who are rejected may work for competitors, may be your customers, or may talk to other candidates. What is it you hope they think and say about your organization and how they were treated?
3. Turn on hospitality and enthusiasm. You do not get a second chance to make a good first impression! Pour enthusiasm into the scene. Your bearing communicates this quickly and effectively. WALK TALL.
4. Meet the candidate in the human resources department. Be on time. Greet him or her by name. When you introduce yourself include your title. Thank the candidate for coming. Offer a rest stop or coffee. Escort him or her to your office.
5. Conduct the interview in privacy. Avoid positioning any furniture between you and the interviewee. Place the person next to your desk rather than across from you. Honor his or her "personal space." Sit erect and lean toward the person. Maintain relatively equal eyelevel. Do not sit on the edge of your desk.
6. Use your very best active listening skill. The candidate should do over 75% of the talking up to the time of your sales pitch.
7. Provide a tour of your facilities. Show off the pleasant environment, efficient arrangements, modern equipment, and access to other departments and facilities.
   Point out that the personnel smile a lot and do not seem harassed. Introduce the candidate to one or two key people, but do not overdo the introductions.
8. Match what the job offers with what the candidate wants. Focus on any special features that are attractive to the person. Use the position description as a guide. If the person has indicated a special interest, eg, in research or teaching, discuss what you have to offer. Create a positive picture in the candidate's mind.
9. Do not forget spouses. Frequently they cast the deciding vote. It is wise to have the candidate's husband or wife sit in on part of the meeting. How does he or she feel about the community and the job opportunity? Is he or she also looking for new employment? What can you offer or suggest?

10. Answer the candidate's questions completely and honestly. Do not conceal negative aspects of the job. Refer to these aspects as challenges. On the other hand, do not dwell on the bad features or say that it has been difficult to keep people in that slot.

11. Avoid salary negotiations until you make an offer. If the person expects more than you offer, keep the door open. Say that you will give more thought to it and report back.[9]

OBTAINING REFERENCES

Remember that an employee may fail in one position and star in another. Get references from more than one job. Obviously, the job that most resembles the one being offered is the most important.

Personal references generally are useless unless they include previous immediate supervisors. The latter are much better sources of information than are senior managers or human resource departments.

Get permission. The application form should contain language whereby applicants grant permission to contact former employers. If not, get this written permission at the time of the interview.

Most currently employed people will not oblige. Abide by that. However, if that person turns out to be the best candidate, make the job offer contingent upon receiving a satisfactory reference from his or her employer. Another strategy is to ask for a copy of candidate's last performance appraisal in lieu of the reference.

Because of the fear of litigation many employers will refuse to comply, will limit responses to dates of employment, or will refuse to confirm data supplied by the applicants. These barriers are not insurmountable. Most reference sources will talk to you if you use the right approach.

How to Conduct a Telephone Reference Check

Here are some practical guidelines provided by Stanton.[10]

1. Make sure you have permission to make the calls.
2. Make the calls yourself. Colleagues are more likely to talk to you than to a human resources clerk.
3. Begin by verifying the information provided by the applicant. After introducing yourself, state "I'd like to verify some information given to us by Ms _____."
   Merely asking for confirmation of information usually elicits a positive response. Ask if this is a good time and place to talk. The person may want to go to another site for more privacy, or may want you to call back later.

   If the person is reluctant to say more, or states that it is against company policy to furnish such information, respond by saying that the lack of information probably will exclude the candidate from further consideration for the job. Ask if an exception can not be made in this case. If that fails, ask to speak to someone at a higher management level.

4. Use some of the same questions you asked the candidate, especially those that relate directly to customer satisfaction. This has the added advantage of evaluating the veracity of the applicant.
5. Follow with more sensitive questions after assuring the respondent that the information will not be revealed to the applicant.
6. Be sensitive to HOW respondents talk about the employee. Are they enthusiastic or brief and guarded?

NOTIFICATION

Do not wait too long before offering the job (24 hours is usually too short, and a month is too long). Tell the candidate how much time he or she has to respond. Notify your top choice first and wait for that person's response before notifying the others. The job offer is usually made in a formal letter from your human resources department. It may be preceded by a telephone call.

REFERENCES

1. Smart B: *The Smart Interviewer.* New York, John Wiley & Sons, 1989.
2. Davidow WB, Uttal B: *Total Customer Service: The Ultimate Weapon.* New York, Harper & Row, 1989.
3. Goldzimer LS: *'I'm First': Your Customer's Message to You.* New York, Rawson Associates, 1989.
4. Perry L: Recruitment materials can impede hiring of nurses. *Mod Healthcare* Jan 20, 1989, p 41.
5. Umiker W: Upgrade your hiring process with this questionnaire. *MLO* 1988;20:37–39.
6. Dortch CT: Job-person match. *Personnel J* 1989;68:48–57.
7. Swan WS: *How to Pick the Right People.* New York, John Wiley & Sons, 1989.
8. Fear R: *The Evaluative Interview.* New York, McGraw-Hill, 1984.
9. Half R: *Half on Hiring.* New York, Crown Publishing, 1985.
10. Stanton ES: Telephone reference checks. *Personnel J* 1988;67:123–130.

9. Indoctrination of New Employees

T HERE ARE THREE considerations in the design of an improved indoctrination program. The first is to orient new employees toward better customer service. The second is to regard the newcomers as clients since they are the recipients of our training services. The third is to infuse the latest concepts of quality assurance. In this chapter we will concentrate on the first two objectives.

Michael Rindler,[1] an outstanding hospital CEO who is known for his expertise in customer service, recommends that the following five values be inculcated as soon as possible: (1) honesty, (2) pride, (3) work ethic, (4) communication, and (5) customer service.

It is hard to find fault with this list, but one can challenge "customer service" as a separate entity since all of the other values also affect customer service. Rindler provides neat examples for each of these values. Honesty means not calling in sick when one is not. Pride is demonstrated in personal appearance and the neatness of work areas. Work ethic is reflected in punctuality and not abusing breaks. Communication is knocking on patient's doors before entering; it is not calling patients "honey" or "dearie." Customer service is going the extra mile, not only for patients, but also for visitors and relatives.

THE SIX OBJECTIVES OF A GOOD ORIENTATION PROGRAM

1. To create a favorable second impression of the organization, the department, and you. The first impression was made at the time of the preemployment interview.
2. To satisfy indoctrinees' need to be accepted by coworkers.

On day 1 make newcomers feel like honored guests. By the second week make them members of your lab family.

3. To establish rapport through collegial communication.
4. To provide initial experiences that result in early successes. This creates a sense of self-value, instills confidence, and promotes positive attitudes. Most athletic coaches like to begin their season against weaker teams for that same reason.
5. To identify all of the laboratory's clients and to emphasize the importance of satisfying them.
6. To initiate the newcomers into the rites and rituals of your quality assurance program.

THE GOLDEN OPPORTUNITY

Kirby[2] puts it well when she writes that we seldom hire "new people." They are usually "used people." Maybe in their past jobs they were not led well. You may be able to turn a marginal employee into a star.

At no other time is there a better opportunity to open lines of communication than with newly hired persons. They are free from the influence of peer groups, they have not yet formed strong opinions about the job, company or boss, and they are so eager to please.[3]

Your goal is to help trainees see their jobs as contributing to the organization's total impact on the customer.[4]

Ten Important Assumptions

Corning Glass Works designed a new orientation system based on the following assumptions[5]:

1. Early impressions last.
2. The first 90 days are crucial.
3. Orientation starts with prearrival activities.
4. Day 1 is crucial.
5. The new employee is responsible for learning.
6. Teaching the basics comes first.
7. New employees should understand the total company.
8. Information is timed to employees' needs.
9. Informational overload must be avoided.
10. Orientation does not work unless the employee's supervisor is involved.

THE HOSPITAL ORIENTATION PROGRAM

New employees are usually enrolled in a hospital orientation program that is directed by the educational department or the human resources department. Most programs start with the history, mission, and philosophy of the organization, but attendees would rather hear about things that affect their job survival, such as opportunities for educational support and other benefits, where to park, when the snack shop opens, and what the ground rules are. Other topics may include information about fires, disasters, safety, infection control, and resuscitation procedures. All too often the orientees are sound asleep by the time these topics are presented.

Departmental Programs

The conceptualization and implementation of a departmental program starts with an analysis of what is needed. The assessments take into account future as well as current requirements. Both the planning and the implementation phases may be slighted because of the time involved and the fact that new arrivals come on board when the department is understaffed—that is why they were hired.

New employees arrive loaded with questions. Planning is facilitated by addressing the following questions even though they may not be articulated.[6]

What are my duties?

How do I answer the phone, order supplies, operate the intercom and all those other things? How well must the work be done? How will I know if I'm doing OK?

When do I come and go? When is payday? When does my probationary period end? When are breaks?

Who does what? Whom do I report to? Who will answer my questions, evaluate my work, be my friend?

Where is my work station, the cafeteria, the restroom, the parking area?

Why do I have to do these things? Why do we do it that way?

Preparations

1. Send a letter of welcome to indoctrinees. Include verification of date, time, and place of reporting, the first day's agenda, and any special instructions or suggestions such as what they should bring or wear.
2. Prepare an orientation packet that includes:
   departmental philosophy, mission statement, and goals
   laboratory organization chart
   position description
   personnel policy and procedures manual
   orientation and training schedules
   checklists and program evaluation forms
   performance appraisal forms
   probationary evaluation form (if it is not same as the performance appraisal form)
   safety, infection control, and quality assurance policies, procedures, and rules
   names, titles and locations of trainers
   key telephone numbers or condensed telephone directory

3. Arrange your schedule so you can devote most of the first day to the orientee.
4. Review the orientation and training check lists.
5. Prepare an agenda for the first week.

THE FIRST DAY OF ORIENTATION

New employees usually report first to the human resources department.[7] Get off to a good start by meeting your new people there: you are the Welcome Wagon. Greet them as you would welcome visiting friends. Offer them coffee and the use of a restroom.

The Attitude and Planning Talk

Have a well-prepared speech and deliver it with enthusiasm. Here is an example:

"Lucy, one of the reasons we selected you is that you seem to have the kind of attitude we look for. As you know, the major goal of this position is to meet or exceed customer expectations. Customers include patients, patient's families and visitors, clinicians and other care providers, third-party payers, teammates, students and trainees, and hospital departments served by the laboratory.

Lucy, I know that you understand the importance of customer service, and know how to deliver it. You're obviously not allergic to work or to changes, and in your past jobs, you demonstrated the flexibility and innovativeness we like in our teammates.

We share your pride in client service. Many members of our medical staff compare our service favorably with that of other labs. Our productivity, as measured by CAP standards is above average, and our lab charges are reasonable."

Explain how each job has a chain reaction with other staff members' ability to do their jobs and therefore eventually affects the customer.[4] Review the first week's agenda and give the new employee his or her indoctrination packet. Get the orientee started. Use the checklists in the orientation packet.

The "Nuts and Bolts" Talk

On the second day, ask how the first day went.[7] Then review together the employee's position description and performance standards. Refer to these documents as contracts that must be honored. Then discuss "survival information" such as work hours, overtime, compensatory time, vacation and sick leave policies, and completing personnel data.

Now is a good time to describe some of the other things you like and dislike. Tell the person how you want to be addressed, whether formally or on a first-name basis. Indicate that you expect everyone to be innovative, that your door is always open, that you welcome suggestions and insist on hearing about any complaints or comments from clients. Say "in this lab we do not kill the messengers of bad tidings."

Mention the things that bug you, such as people slipping in a little late each day, untidy clothes, or verbal expressions such as "that's not in my position description" or "I only work here." It's better to prevent what you do not like, than to have to correct it after the fact.

Hochheiser[8] recommends that you promise new employees that you will do as much as you can to help them meet their goals if they will obey the following five rules:

1. They will be loyal to you at all times.
2. They will help you look good.
3. They will not go over your head to change your directives.
4. They will cooperate with one another.
5. They will acknowledge that only one hero is allowed in the group, and that is you.

Show and Tell Time

Do not try to cover everything during a single tour of the premises—that is too confusing for new employees. Avoid information overload. But do point out the physical facilities. Do not stop repeatedly to introduce all of the personnel. You will do this later.

On a subsequent tour, follow the sequences of various work flows. For example, trace a test request from its point of origin to the posting of results. Instruct the indoctrinees to diagram these work flows. Show how customer service is affected by glitches in these work flows.

Devote one session to a discussion of budgets, charges, and laboratory costs. Orientees should be shown how charges appear on patient's bills, and how they can respond to customers' questions about them.

Direct attention to the communication systems, and demonstrate their use. Stress the importance of proper telephone etiquette. (This subject is so important that a separate chapter is devoted to it.) Include the intercom, bulletin boards, mailboxes and message centers. Point out where schedules for work, off-duty assignments, and vacations are posted. Show them how the different shifts communicate with each other. Demonstrate how photocopying and filing are done. The location and use of safety equipment are best covered separately.

Some laboratory managers arrange for trainees to make rounds with physicians and to attend meetings of the nursing staffs and medical staff committees. The importance of maintaining cordial relations with the nurses is stressed, and the trainees should be reminded that nurses are clients of the laboratory.

After the tours have been completed, ask the new people to diagram the topography of the department. This should include the labeling of each room. Later, have them draw more detailed diagrams of the room(s) to which they are assigned, and to locate on these drawings each work station and major piece of equipment.

Meeting Coworkers

I recommend against a lot of introductions during the laboratory tours. Employees do not like to be interrupted in the middle of tasks, and this may be misinterpreted by the orientees as unfriendliness. Also, the new folks get confused by all the faces, names, and titles when presented in rapid succession.

Make the introductions during breaks, when people are relaxed and more inclined to be amiable. Also present newcomers at a staff meeting. Encourage them to talk about their educational and recreational interests at that time.

When you introduce someone, indicate how that person's responsibilities or interests relate to the newcomer. An introduction might go like this: "Joyce, I'd like you to meet Sue Smith. Sue is in charge of our main storeroom. If you can't find something there, see Sue."

The new employee should meet with each senior member of the laboratory staff, preferably in his or her office.

The Trainer or Educational Coordinator

If you delegate the training, have the new employee meet the trainer early in the orientation program. Pick trainers with care. Prerequisites include teaching ability, professional or technical expertise, sufficient time, willingness, and loads of enthusiasm.

Trainers should be aware of the qualifications and experience of the indoctrinees so they can tailor the training to the particular needs of each individual. The orientee's supervisor should also participate in this planning process.

Trainees may be given folders in which to keep their continuing education records. Most laboratories have requirements for a minimal number of hours annually for each job category. The trainees are instructed on how these records should be kept, and reminded that it is their responsibility to do so.

The Safety Coordinator

Many laboratories have a manager or technologist who is a specialist in safety and preventive medicine. This person often serves on the hospital infection control committee. The safety coordinator shows newly hired persons the location and proper use of safety equipment, and reviews the safety policies and regulations. Topics include sites where eating and smoking are permitted, protective clothing and gloves, handling of contaminated specimens and work surfaces, and the disposal of needles, broken glass, and other dangerous materials.

New employees often have questions about the dangers of hepatitis, AIDS, and other infectious diseases. The safety expert can allay these fears while demonstrating the best techniques for minimizing such dangers. When discussing AIDS, the expert warns against disclosure of confidential information.

The Laboratory Information Service Specialist

Most laboratories are now computerized, and have at least one staff member who serves as laboratory information service (LIS) instructor and troubleshooter.

The Quality Assurance Coordinator

This person may be chairperson or recorder for the laboratory quality assurance (QA) committee. The QA coordinator may limit his or her discussions to the global aspects of the QA program, leaving specific quality control details for the orientee's immediate supervisor.

Mentors and "Buddies"

Mentors are experienced professionals or managers who willingly share their wisdom or political clout with their proteges. They are unofficial advisors, supporters, and confidants. New employees are encouraged to establish alliances with these individuals.

In some laboratories, the "buddy system" is used. Each new arrival is assigned to an experienced employee in the same work section.

THE TRAINING OF NEW EMPLOYEES

"Training is the secret of cost-effective staffing and a cornerstone of customer satisfaction."[4]

"Vestibule" training is the final education new employees receive before being turned loose. Training is aimed not only at building skills, but also at instilling healthy mental attitudes. Teaching a clerk how to answer the telephone is skills training. Teaching that person how to please callers, is part of attitude development. Positive attitude tends to piggyback on skill improvement.

Without special training the bonding necessary for customer satisfaction is left to chance. Customer service skills, like technical skills, are acquired.[14] For training to take, the first-line supervisor must know what is being taught and reward, reinforce, and support the new behaviors.[4]

Strike a balance between social and technical training. Do not forget the internal customers. Cross train to increase employees' abilities to solve customer problems on their own.

Preparations by Trainer

1. Review the position description and resume of the trainee.
2. Prepare a checklist of procedures to be learned.
3. Identify teaching methods to be used.
4. Prepare teaching aids including equipment, specimens, lists of questions, handouts, and references.
5. Check notes. Update if necessary.

6. Prepare a daily teaching agenda.
7. Make certain that a classroom or benchwork area is available.
8. Make necessary changes in the daily routine to allow sufficient time for the trainees.

Stimulating Creativity in Trainees

As newcomers become familiar with your procedures, they will compare your equipment, methods, and practices with those of previous employers, or with what they were taught during their internships. Trainers who are self-confident and know how to encourage innovation will not only accept well-intentioned criticism, they will invite questions and comments. You do not want preceptors who slough off suggestions with remarks like "just do it our way and you'll get along fine," "that would never work here," or "that's a rather stupid idea." These comments are creativity destroyers, especially when uttered sarcastically. Unfortunately, creativity is often sacrificed for conformity during the training process.

Praise-Criticism Ratio

A common weakness of bench work instruction is the tendency to be generous with criticism but stingy with praise. Well-meaning preceptors, concentrating on correcting faulty techniques, often point out only the things that trainees do wrong. There are lots of exclamations like, "No, not that way. Let me show you again." A common complaint from trainees is that they only get negative feedback. Actually, there are abundant opportunities to praise performance. Even the technologist who is all thumbs does most things right.

There are two simple techniques that are helpful. The first is to maintain a positive praise-criticism ratio. At the end of a learning session, reflect on the comments you have issued. How many were positive and how many were negative? By paying attention to this ratio you will find that you increase the number of positives. You become a better supporter, and your charges respond with more enthusiasm.

The second method is the "enhancing value" technique. When a procedural error or cognitive lapse is noted, the trainer says, "Sue, I like the way you prepared the specimens and ran the standards. [At this point avoid the word "but."] I think that if you would . . . you'd be operating that machine as well as the rest of us." The first part of that statement lets Sue know that you are her supporter. Now she's more receptive to the criticism that follows. The last part of the statement, like the first, promotes self-esteem.

Six Tips for Better Training

1. Plan a highly structured process. The trainee should know what is to be learned each day, who will do the instructing, and how to prepare for the next day's work. Use an outline for each learning segment.
2. Develop a success habit by working on easier skills first.

3. Correct errors before they become habits, but do not nitpick.
4. Address errors, not traits or personality. Regard errors as learning experiences.
5. Expect to have to repeat things. Avoid that exasperated facial expression when you do.
6. Treat trainees as knowledgeable adults.

"Graduation"

A good indoctrination program requires much mental effort and psychological stress on the part of trainees. Therefore, the last day should be a special one for them. Three events are appropriate:

1. The supervisor meets with them to:
   review the checklists and critiques to ensure that everything has been covered.
   schedule any incomplete or omitted activities.
   discuss any last minute problems or trainee's suggestions
   congratulate them.
2. The department chief meets with them. Before this meeting, the chief reviews all of the indoctrination reports and meets with the "faculty." At this meeting, members of the group point out needs for additional experience, behaviors to watch out for, and special accomplishments or attributes that have been manifested, eg, "Steve made several helpful suggestions, for example . . . .". The boss likes to be able to say something complimentary and specific to show that he or she knows what's going on. Also, favorable comments from the top brass carry added weight. They indicate to the trainee that favorable reports do go up the chain of command.
3. Celebrate the event at the next staff meeting. The boss makes a nice speech and the trainees take their bows and revel in the applause (it may be the last they receive for a long time). Thank all the staffers who helped. Encourage the trainees to voice their appreciation. Make sure that no one has been excluded. You may be surprised at how many people helped.

The Follow-Up

Evaluate the program by holding frequent informal chats with the indoctrinees and your fellow trainers. At a formal interview held upon completion of the program, document data for the probationary report.

Some laboratory managers like to give a written quiz to orientees. This has merit. It may reveal deficiencies on the part of the trainee, or the program. In either instance, additional action is needed before the trainee is turned loose on the customers. In any event, written critiques by trainees are important. Surveys taken several months after trainees have been performing their new duties long enough to be able to pass judgment on the training they received are even more valuable.

REFERENCES

1. Rindler M: *Putting Patients and Profits Into Perspective*. Chicago, Pluribus Press, 1987.
2. Kirby T: *The Can-do Manager*. New York, AMACOM, 1989.
3. Werther WB Jr: *Dear Boss*. New York, Meadowbrook Press, 1989.
4. Goldzimer LS: *'I'm First': Your Customer's Message to You*. New York, Rawson Associates, 1989.
5. Ideas and trends in personnel. *Hum Resources Manage* July 26, 1988.
6. Reinhardt C: Training supervisors in first-day orientation techniques. *Personnel* 1988;65:24–28.
7. Umiker W: *Management Skills for the New Health Care Supervisor*. Rockville, MD, Aspen Publishers Inc, 1988.
8. Hochheiser RM: *How to Work for a Jerk*. New York, Vintage Books, 1987.

10. Performance Reviews and Rewards

MPLOYEES ARE EVALUATED and rewarded on the basis of how well they meet the performance standards stipulated in their position descriptions. In a previous chapter we described how to introduce customer expectations into position descriptions and work standards.

EMPLOYEES ARE BOTH SERVICE PROVIDERS AND CUSTOMERS

When employees are regarded as customers, the appraisal system must permit employees to evaluate their superiors and tell them how they can be more effective leaders ("bottom-up" or "reverse" performance appraisals).

As service providers to employee-customers, supervisors and managers use formal and informal work reviews to help their employees reach their full potential, to help them design new objectives, to help them to implement their action plans, and to provide psychological support.

An organization that features customer satisfaction is not achieved by proclaiming dedication to service, nor by issuing lofty mission statements in the hope that customers will believe them and that the fine words will trickle down the hierarchy. Excellence in service is achieved only when proclamations are translated into things discernible to the customer. [1] Every employee must accept the concept, commit to it, and know precisely what is expected of him or her and, conversely, what rewards can be expected.

Designing an Appraisal/Reward Strategy

1. Find out what clients want.

2. Set standards.
3. Measure performance against these standards.
4. Devise a system that rewards the desired performance.[1]

FEEDBACK: THE BREAKFAST OF CHAMPIONS[2]

We have already discussed how to find out what customers want and how to incorporate those wants into position descriptions and work standards. These changes in the position descriptions are reinforced during performance reviews. Appraisal interviews provide ideal opportunities for the supervisor and the interviewee to develop explicit objectives and plans for better customer service.[3]

Measuring performance against new standards is not easy because many customer-service descriptors are highly subjective ("soft data"). Combine this problem with that of a pay-for-performance reward system and you open the door to charges of discrimination or favoritism, largely because many customer input systems are flawed. For example, the "comment cards" found in motels and restaurants are usually filled out only by patrons who are either very pleased or very dissatisfied. More reliable feedback requires surveys, focus groups, frequent meetings with selected customers; or including clients in planning sessions, quality circles, training exercises and orientation programs. Employers, realizing the limitations of anecdotal evidence, are moving toward formalizing the survey process.[1]

More reliable use of (and return from) feedback requires regular application. The most powerful input is derived from day-to-day coaching. To rely entirely on an annual performance review is equivalent to using a single examination to determine whether a student passes or fails.

WHAT GETS REWARDED GETS DONE

The closer the connection between customer satisfaction and the rewards to employees, the greater the likelihood of customer satisfaction.[4] Here is a personal vignette that brought this home to me. I, like other Americans, was accustomed to poor automobile service by dealers. When I picked up my most recently purchased car (Toyota), I found an unusual note on the front seat. Instead of the usual promise of outstanding service, it simply asked that on each service visit I fill out a thorough customer-satisfaction form "because the salaries and bonuses of our service manager and his assistants are determined mostly by how satisfied you are." Thus far, service has been truly outstanding.

The rewards can be the same as those for any other kind of good performance, including bonuses, salary increases, promotions, special awards, and recognition. Yet nothing is more effective than earned praise from a leader who is highly respected.

Pitfalls in Appraisal Interviews

The review is used to distribute salary increases instead of to improve performance.

The meeting is conducted as a lecture rather than as an interview.
The supervisor does all the talking.
Lack of or outdated objectives.
Inadequate preparation by manager or employee.
The evaluation is highly subjective.
Emphasis is on the past rather than on the future.

The Four Essentials of Performance Reviews

(1) Review and clarify what you expect based on job descriptions, work standards, and performance objectives. (2) Evaluate the performance. (3) Express your appreciation for the employee's accomplishments, behavior, and effort. (4) Plan (this is the most important segment).

A good review combines the features of recognition, self-appraisal, joint problem-solving, and management by objectives. Emphasis is on the future rather than on the past. Planning is stressed over evaluation. The review makes employees feel like winners and that is its most important feature.

Success breeds success. A little of it makes us want to do even better. Expressions of appreciation and commendations are more effective than criticism, however constructive and well-intentioned the latter is. Studies have shown that performance usually decreases after criticism. Therefore, it makes sense to spend more time delivering positive strokes than harping on deficiencies. Use prior counseling sessions to deal with performance problems.

PREPARING FOR PERFORMANCE REVIEW INTERVIEWS

As for any meeting, advance planning is the key to success. The meeting has two components, the process and the content. The process consists of the format and the interviewer's skill. The content is what transpires during the meeting.

Get Employee Input

The employee should have the following documents:

a position description, including performance standards.
the evaluation form used to report the review.
a copy of the last formal review.
instructions on how to prepare for the meeting.
departmental objectives for the current year.

Employees may be asked to fill out the evaluation form and give it to the interviewer before the meeting (self-appraisal). The employee should prepare a list of objectives and plans relating to improvement needs and career development, including specific requests for assistance needed to achieve the new objectives. The employee should also record a list of what he or she regards as significant contributions made to the department, and activities that gave the most satisfactions.

Review the Employee's Personnel File

Personnel records should include the following: a position description and standards of performance; continuing education and attendance records; commendations, special recognition, or awards; incident reports, and records of counseling or disciplinary actions; a report of the last review.

Review New Department Objectives

You want to synchronize the employee's objectives with those of your department, with new emphasis on customer satisfaction.

Discuss Performance With Other Observers

Other observers may include managers to whom the person reports or individuals who work with the person.

Prepare an Agenda

Set a date, time, and place. Give the employee sufficient time to prepare for the meeting. Set aside at least an hour for the interview.

Formulate Key Remarks

Select the exact words to use for introductory statements, to criticize, and to confront defensiveness. Avoid the word "average" (everyone thinks he or she is above average). Anticipate problems. Be ready to cite specific examples to illustrate your points.

Make Necessary Changes in Your Interview Procedure

You may want to add items to appraisal forms. If your organization still uses rating forms based exclusively on traits and nonspecific behavior (honesty, loyalty, quantity and quality of work, and the like), add behavior criteria that relate directly to duties and responsibilities documented in position descriptions.

Many organizations use the same form for all categories of employees and for all hierarchic levels. These forms often lack rating factors pertaining to administrative and supervisory responsibilities. If you evaluate individuals who serve in leadership roles, add these factors. Another appropriate addition is a record of the degree of success in achieving objectives formulated at previous performance reviews. Last, and not at all least, introduce indicators relating to quality assurance and customer satisfaction.

Why You Should Avoid Discussing
Salary at This Meeting

Once salary talk is introduced, it dominates and distorts the discussion. Even worse, it incites an adversarial relationship. Instead of accepting higher work standards or more challenging objectives, employees argue for lower ones. Also, if the employee is told that no monetary reward is forthcoming, the resulting resentment can prevent a freewheeling discussion of new objectives and plans.

Be prepared to respond if an employee should press for a discussion of salary adjustments. Reply that while performance ratings are important, other factors affect salary. These factors include the employee's new objectives, the availability and market value of certain categories, what competitors are paying, and budget constraints. Tell the employee that he or she will be informed later when the information is available. Discuss this at a subsequent brief meeting. If it is absolutely necessary to discuss salary at the performance review, save it for last.

STEPS IN THE PERFORMANCE REVIEW AND PLANNING INTERVIEW

The three segments of a performance review and planning interview are as follows:

Update the position description.
Discuss past performance and fill out the appraisal form.
Discuss future performance.

Update the Position Description

Position descriptions provide the underpinning for effective performance appraisals. Therefore, these informal contracts should be addressed first. Add quality assurance and client-satisfaction descriptors if this has not already been done.

Duties and Responsibilities

The following questions provide a nonthreatening, job-focused opening:

Are you performing any duties not listed in your position description?
What more would you like to be responsible for?
What are you doing that you think should be done by someone else?
What assignments do you find most enjoyable? Least enjoyable?

Standards of Performance

Does the person understand and accept these?
Should any be added or changed?

Range of Authority

Has lack of authority been a barrier to performance?
Has the right to more freedom of action been earned?

Discuss Past Performance and Complete the Appraisal Form

Follow the instructions of your human resources department, but do not limit yourself to these guidelines.

Self-Appraisal

The concept of self-appraisal says to the subordinate: "Your input is important." Most employees rate themselves the same as or below what their bosses do. Only a few have inflated self-opinions and they seldom accept their boss' opinion on anything.[5]

Discuss Ratings

Review any customer ratings, commendatory reports, incident reports, and complaints pertaining to the ratee. These should be given substantial weight in the rating process.

When self-evaluation is included, cover issues in the following order.

1. Highly rated items on which you and the employee agree. This is based on the principle that you must start with something positive. If you begin with something negative, the person will not hear what follows.
2. Low rating by employee . . . you disagree.
3. Low rating . . . both of you agree.
4. Higher rating by employee . . . you disagree.

(**A caveat:** The most common and serious error is to overrate marginal performers. Overrating often returns to haunt managers.)

Note: When people dispute your ratings, listen carefully to their complaints. Do not become defensive. Permit them to write dissenting opinions.

Commendatory comments should include the following elements:

A statement that performance exceeded expectations.
Description of the specific contribution by the person.
The beneficial effects to the organization that resulted from the employee's action.
Your congratulations and appreciation.
How the performance will be rewarded (if appropriate).

How to Criticize

Criticism must be palatable but substantial. Preserving self-esteem does not mean being lenient. Concentrate on output or results when possible. Otherwise, address behavior, or the need to improve qualifications relating to knowledge, skill, or experience. Avoid the word "attitude" as much as possible. When you must use it, be prepared to give examples.

Never attack the ratee. Join forces in attacking the problem. Ask poor performers what they think the effects of their continued behavior will be. Get them to focus on the consequences of their actions.[6]

Communication Tips

Figure 10.1 provides some suggestions for better communication during appraisal interviews. Listening skill deserves special attention. Active listening is listening in which you reassure speakers that you got the right message, and also that you understand their feelings about that message. Practice active listening using the following special techniques:

1. Attending, ie, paying attention to eye contact, facial expression, voice tone, and body language.
2. Using door openers, such as "I'd like to hear more about that."
3. Reflecting, which involves the use of expletives such as "I see . . . Uh-huh . . . go on" to indicate that you are listening. These utterances are accompanied by head nodding.
4. Responding techniques:
   "I can understand why you're upset" (empathic response).
   "Give me an example" (probing response).
   "Our policy is . . ." (explanatory response).
   "I think you're saying" (summarizing response).
5. Silence really is golden when you are trying to draw an employee out. Count to ten or wait until the silence becomes uncomfortable.

Discuss Future Performance

Over half of the interview should be devoted to a discussion of the future. Again, past performance should always provide the database for planning future activities.

Improvement Needs

There is little chance for improvement unless there is agreement that improvement is needed and possible. This agreement is arrived at only after honest dialogue. This is the most sensitive part of the interview, so tread lightly. Remember that your goal is to help the employee reach full potential. Focus on those things that are directly observed by you or are reliably reported to you.

Use a directive approach when you want to reinforce desired behavior: "Your monthly progress reports are excellent. Don't change a thing!" When dealing with a performance problem, use a nondirective approach: "What can we do to get those reports out on time every month?"

Use "I" instead of "You" language when finding fault: "I still get complaints about turnaround time" is better than "You must do something about turn-around time." Use "You" language when praising.

Let the employee do most of the talking.

Use your best listening skill.

Give examples:
"I would feel better if you volunteered more often for special assignments."

Do not be controlling. Do not try to force the person to your point of view. Accept his or her lack of agreement as a right.

Do not give unsolicited advice:
"If I were you . . ." is seldom appreciated and usually goes unheeded.

Do not erode the employee's self-esteem. Do not ridicule, kid, or call names. Anything that starts with "The trouble with you is . . ." is destructive.

Figure 10.1 Suggestions for better dialogues.

Discuss New Objectives

Employees who leave an appraisal session without new work objectives and an action plan are being shortchanged. Open this segment by enlightening them on departmental changes that may affect their objectives.

Objectives are powerful motivational tools, but like all tools, they must be used properly. The objectives must be attainable. If a person has an 80% chance of achieving an objective, it will be challenging. If the chance is 50% or less, the objective will be incapacitating.[7]

When employees have difficulty in articulating objectives, simply ask them what they think needs to be done. Another useful tactic is for the rater to state three things he or she would like to see improved, and have the ratee mention three things the rater could do, or stop doing, to help.

The characteristics of good objectives can be expressed in the acronym SCRAM.

Specific
Challenging
Relevant
Achievable
Measurable

For each objective each party should answer the following questions:

1. *What* is my goal? What is to be done? What will I be? or What will I have?
   "I will improve my listening skill." *or*
   "I'm going to be a better listener." *or*
   "I will have better rapport with complainers."

Answer telephone within 3 rings

Cross train in another laboratory section

Serve as mentor for new employee

Serve on committee or quality circle

Increase number of lab bulletins for medical staff

Present monthly talk to nursing staff

Set up quality control system for physician's office labs

Teach bedside lab techniques to nursing staff

Spend 1 day per month at a nursing station

Attend medical grand rounds once each quarter

Design a recording system for customer complaints

Attend a seminar on telephone use

Reorganize the orientation program

Visit emergency room, special care units, and surgical suite monthly

Design a questionnaire to survey physician satisfaction

Complete performance appraisals on time

Reduce turnaround time by 10%

Learn Spanish to improve patient communication

Devise a system to eliminate unnecessary screens

Revise lab request and report forms

Figure 10.2   Examples of customer service objectives.

2. *Why* do I want this goal?
   "I'll learn more about what needs to be done to improve customer service."
3. *How* will I do this?
   "I'll enroll in at least one communication seminar, read one book and at least five articles on listening skill, and practice this skill at work and at home."
4. *Who* must I get to help?
5. *When* will I start? When is the first follow-up date?

List any serious obstacles to attaining a particular goal and how best to overcome them.

Techniques to ensure success:

1. Limit the number of objectives.
2. Select objectives that are attainable.
3. Put them in writing.
4. Discuss them with at least one other person in addition to your boss.
5. Use a follow-up sheet and make weekly progress entries.

What factors favor success?

What or who represents constraints?

How is this to be funded?

Who else must approve the plan?

Who else will help carry out the plan?
- Are they aware of their role?
- Are they able and willing to help?

Whom do I check with on my progress, and when?

Do I have a realistic timetable?

What indicators can I use to monitor progress?

What reports must be prepared?

Is there a backup plan?

Figure 10.3 Performance objectives are hollow statements without action plans. These questions are helpful in thinking through such plans.

(**A caveat:** Don't accept "I'll try." When people say that, they are building excuses for failure. If they fail, they claim that they did what they said they would . . . try.[6])

See Figure 10.2 for a list of possible objectives relating to customer satisfaction. Performance objectives are hollow statements without plans. Figure 10.3 presents questions that are helpful in thinking through such plans.

End the Interview on a Positive Note: Summarize Key Points

Reassure and express confidence in the interviewee and thank him or her for cooperating. Schedule follow-up sessions, if necessary, to cover salary discussion, remedial counseling, career counseling, detailed planning, or progress in meeting objectives. Do not wait for the next formal review.

(**A caveat:** Never add negative comments after the employee has signed off.)

"BOTTOM-UP" PERFORMANCE APPRAISALS

Let us return to our employees as customers. As in the case of other customer services, it is a mistake to rely on complaints and grievances to detect supervisors and managers who are not performing up to par. Only a small percentage of employees will lodge official gripes. Detection of the "bad apples" is often complicated by the fact that their "numbers" may look good over the short haul. By the time signs such as high turnover, absenteeism, and grievances surface, irreparable damage may have been inflicted. Employers can no longer wait that long.

Progressive organizations do not hesitate to conduct opinion surveys among their employees. Unfortunately most of these do not pinpoint problems with specific managers.[8] Employee surveys are now being supplemented by formal bottom-up appraisals in which subordinates anonymously rate their bosses. These appraisals provide information that helps to detect and solve morale and productivity problems.

Rating factors are determined by what employees are capable of evaluating. Employees at the lower organizational levels are usually unfamiliar with financial and strategic concepts.[8] Appropriate raters are those who have frequent and significant contact with the ratee. Usually, these are the people who are rated by the manager.[8]

Managers' resistance to this process is the greatest barrier. They rationalize that the ratings may be based on popularity rather than respect. This has apparently not been a problem at organizations where this strategy was actually implemented.[8]

REFERENCES

1. Lee C: Using customers' ratings to reward employees. *Training* 1989;26:40–46.

2. Blanchard K, Lorb R: *Putting the One-Minute Manager to Work*. New York, William Morrow Co, 1984.

3. Cocheu T: Refocus performance objectives toward greater customer service. *Personnel J* 1988;4:116–120.

4. LeBoeuf M: *The Greatest Management Principle in the World*. New York, Berkley Books, 1985.

5. Locher AH, Teel KS: Appraisal trends. *Personnel J* 1988;67:139–145.

6. Werther WB Jr: *Dear Boss*. New York, Meadowbrook Press, 1989.

7. Hochheiser RM: *How to Work for a Jerk*. New York, Vintage Books, 1987.

8. Nevels P: Why employees are being asked to rate their supervisors. *Supervis Manage* 1989;34:5–11.

11. Oral Communication for Service Providers

THE AVERAGE MANAGER spends three times more time talking and listening than writing and reading. Verbal communication skill is the very essence of client relations.

SERVICE PROVIDERS AS SENDERS

To be effective senders, people must command respect. First and foremost, they respect themselves, having confidence, self-esteem, and poise. They exhibit this when their unspoken message to clients is, "I can help you because I'm in the know."

Employers must empower employees who provide the customer contacts, but who are often at the bottom of the table of organization. Turn that table upside down, with customers and the employees who serve them at the top. Management's role is to support these first-line troops by instilling pride and ensuring competence. This involves careful hiring practices, thorough indoctrination, continuous training and coaching, and rewarding of performance excellence.

Empowered employees are not afraid to speak up and make their needs known. When they do not speak up, they are sending the message, "I'm not important."[1]

Workers are in a better position to answer clients' questions when they know what is going on outside their own limited work stations. One of the benefits of cross training and work station rotation is that service providers can respond better to questions and requests from patrons.

Show That We Care

A UCLA psychologist claims that in general verbal communication only 7% of feelings are transmitted by words.[2]

Thirty-eight percent come from how the words are articulated, and 55% are conveyed through body language.

When dealing with customers in general, and patients in particular, feelings are pivotal both in sending and receiving messages. It is crucial for us to know how the customer feels about our service, and, as we have just learned, more than half of that feeling is visually transmitted. We also want our customers to know that we care about them.

Get the Customers' Attention

You only get one chance to make a first impression.

We form impressions of others very quickly, in a matter of seconds, so get off to a fast start. Concentrate on the first 30 seconds, the length of most television advertisements. These 30 seconds are the most important. Keep the dialogue brief out of consideration for the client's time. More than 5 minutes are seldom needed.

1. Grab the client's attention.
   Promise something: "Would you like a faster turnaround time?"
   Praise the client for something done or said.
2. Maintain the client's interest.
   Mention mutual acquaintances, backgrounds, or experience.[2]
   "I understand you trained with . . ."
   "Are you a graduate of Penn State, too?"
   "That's interesting. We had the same problem with that software."
   Use names frequently.
   Ask for opinions: "I need to know how you think we could eliminate that problem."
3. Power up your messages.
   Speak with conviction. Exhibit confidence by word and body. Establish and maintain eye contact. If the person seems uncomfortable with eye contact, glance aside occasionally.
   Speak firmly and clearly, not too fast or too slow. Watch out for robotic monotone.
   Substitute strong for weak responses:
   "Gee, I don't know. I'm not the one to ask. I'll try to find out and get back to you." (weak)
   "That's important and I want to make sure that I give you the right answer. Will you be in your office at 11 o'clock?" (more powerful—you're in control)
   Avoid "weakeners" such as:
   "I feel we would . . ." ("let's . . .")
   "I wonder if you would . . ." ("please send . . .")
   "I'm no expert, but . . ." ("I suggest that . . .")
   "Is there any chance that . . ." ("We'll expect you to . . .OK?")
   Give color and power to your messages by creating imagery, using highly descriptive words, and personalizing messages.

4. Close strongly. State what you will do, or what you want the client to do, if anything.

   "We'll get the new instrument next month."

   "If you get your requests in by . . ."

   "I thought I'd run it by you because it will come up at the next meeting.

When cornered by rambling or long-winded customers, summarize what they said and what you are going to do. Try not to appear impatient as you ask to be excused.

COMMUNICATION BARRIERS

We may have only limited control over ambient distractions such as noise, temperature, humidity, and odors, but we can reduce personal factors such as finger-pointing, scratching, sniffling, jingling, or fidgeting. We often erect two other barriers to effective communication almost without thinking, semantic and psychological.

Semantic

We speak five languages: (1) english; (2) body language; (3) professional and technical jargon; (4) organizational and bureaucratic talk; and (5) computer language.

Consider the educational level of your listeners. An explanation to a physician is quite different from that to a patient who has a limited vocabulary. Even a well-educated client may not be familiar with medical terminology.

Avoid jargon and acronymns unless you know that your listeners understand this language. Euphemisms and other vague or abstract language only confuse. Slang is seldom suitable. Fillers like "ya know . . right on . . ya gotta be kidding" are anathema.

Psychological

These are the most pernicious. They include:

mixed messages. The words do not match the body language.
interrupting.
arguing, blaming, or name-calling.
talking down to, kidding, or being sarcastic.
inflammatory statements such as "You must" or "I demand."
emotional, sexist, or patronizing words, such as "you girls" or "those jerks," must
   be avoided like the plague.

Another pitfall is failure to verify assumptions. We do this all the time. For instance, we say "Do you understand?" The person nods. We say "Do you have any questions?" The person again nods. In both instances we assume that our message has been understood. Maybe it has or maybe it hasn't. If we substitute,

"What questions do you have?" or better still, "I may not have been very clear, what's your understanding of our agreement?" we elicit more definite feedback. Close observation of the person's facial expression also provides clues as to whether the communication has been understood.

SERVICE PROVIDERS AS RECEIVERS

"Mom, you never listen to me."
"My dear husband, please put down that paper and listen to me."
"I tried to explain what was wrong, but the clerk would not listen."

Sound familiar? You bet. Most people are lousy listeners. If you design a customer service program that does nothing more than teach how to listen, it will be worthwhile. Clients will be treated better, and the learners' interpersonal relations will improve.

You can send associates to "smile school" or teach them to maintain eye contact while reciting "have a good day," but if they have not learned how to listen, you have struck out. When customers are confronted by blank smiles and mumbled greetings, they are irritated because what they see and hear is perceived as phony.

Not only must we listen, we must also make certain that the other person knows that we are listening. Test your own listening skill by taking the quiz in Figure 11.1.

The Three Keys to Good Listening

1. Listen for facts.
2. Listen for feelings.
3. Listen with your eyes.

GOOD AND BAD LISTENING RESPONSES

1. Defensive responses (the worst) reveal lack of confidence and self-worth: "That's a lie, and I resent it."
2. Evaluative responses (not much better) are judgmental or critical. They usually start with "you": "You expect too much of us," or "You always find something to complain about."
3. Explanatory responses (OK if wanted by receiver) inform, advise or recommend. Usually bad if the word "policy" is included. Avoid "Our policy does not permit that" or "I'll tell you what you must do."
4. Probing responses (excellent if not overdone) get the information you need. They're questions that deal with "who, where, why, when, what, and how."
5. Empathic responses (the best) are nonjudgmental, supportive responses that reflect feelings. They often make use of paraphrasing: "You're saying that you're not getting the service you deserve. I can understand why that upsets you."

You do:

1. honor his personal space (about 3 feet).   3 2 1
2. focus your eyes steadily on his face.   3 2 1
3. let him complete his sentences.   3 2 1
4. let him express himself completely before you talk.   3 2 1
5. ask open-ended questions.   3 2 1
6. make a special effort to interpret body language.   3 2 1
7. use brief assertions such as "I see" or "Uh-huh."   3 2 1
8. use reflective facial expressions such as smiling, or nodding.   3 2 1
9. paraphrase and reflect his feelings.   3 2 1
10. concentrate on getting the right message.   3 2 1
11. see things from his point of view.   3 2 1
12. emphasize points of agreement.   3 2 1
13. disagree with conviction but without heat.   3 2 1

You avoid or refrain from:

14. thinking of your response while he's still talking.   3 2 1
15. fidgeting with papers or pencil.   3 2 1
16. sneaking glances at your watch.   3 2 1
17. interrupting, even when you know he's wrong or abusive.   3 2 1
18. inserting humorous remarks when he's serious.   3 2 1
19. feigning listening.   3 2 1
20. letting your gaze wander.   3 2 1
21. letting your mind wander.   3 2 1
22. insisting on getting the last word.   3 2 1
23. finishing his sentences.   3 2 1
24. kidding, sarcasm, or put-downs.   3 2 1
25. making inflammatory statements ("You're confused" or "I demand").   3 2 1

Your score:

Figure 11.1 Test your listening skill. 3 indicates usually; 2, occasionally; and 1, seldom. Total your score, but note that there is no magic number. The higher your total score, the less you need to be concerned about your listening skill. Reevaluate yourself at weekly intervals, however.

SUGGESTIONS FOR BETTER LISTENING

1. Use active listening. To the inactive or passive listener, information "goes in one ear and out the other." Active listening is hearing, understanding,

analyzing, and ensuring that you received the right message. Active listening requires energy, so avoid it when you are overtired, especially when the conversation is important.

According to a theory known as neurolinguistic programming, people are divided into three groups according to the primary way in which they perceive their environment.[3] The first group thinks in terms of pictures or images. They use a lot of "eye" language, eg, "I can SEE what you mean." Their eyes move upward when they listen. People in the second group have auditory orientation. They say, "I haven't HEARD anything important." Their eyes move down and to the left. Individuals who perceive things through feelings say, "I FEEL that we're on the right track." Their eyes move down and to the right. It is believed that we communicate better when we mirror these kinds of word reception.

2. Stop listening defensively.

Do not take criticism or complaints personally.

Do not react by counterattacking.

Do not be judgmental ("You're wrong on both counts").

Do ask probing questions ("Please give me more details").

3. Listen for feelings.

People who want us to listen to their problems often do not want solutions, they just want sympathetic listening, even though they say they want your opinion.

A powerful way of establishing rapport is to reflect what you see or hear. If the person seems friendly, respond cheerfully. If she is angry, show concern. If he appears anxious and harried, exhibit urgency.

Use comprehenders like "Uh-huh . . . Go on . . . I understand," accompanied by nods, smiles, or other supporting body language. Open-ended questions are the best conversational door openers. Use periods of silence. They are great for getting the person to open up.

Ten Things to Avoid in Active Listening

1. Trying to listen when you do not have the time.
2. Mental script writing. This is thinking of how you are going to respond when you should be listening.
3. Feigning listening. You can seldom fake it.
4. Interrupting. Either you are not listening, or you are being impolite.
5. Hogging airtime.
6. Making value judgments. Customers hate this.
7. Too much advising or persuading. You are perceived as patronizing.
8. Denying the client's feelings, eg, "You shouldn't feel that way." (Who are you to say how they should feel?)
9. Expressing glib or phony promises. This is the surest way to destroy your credibility.
10. Using put-downs. See Figure 11.2 for examples of "downers."

Don't be ridiculous.

We tried that once before.

It costs too much.

It can't be done.

That's not our responsibility.

That's too radical a change.

We don't have the time.

We've never done that before.

Why change? It's still working okay.

It isn't in the budget.

We're not ready for that.

Let's form a committee.

Let's get back to reality.

We'll be the laughing stock.

We did all right without it.

If it was good, others would be doing it.

If it was good, we would be doing it.

Figure 11.2 Downers.

BODY LANGUAGE

Kinesics is the study of body movements, facial expressions, and gestures as they relate to communication. I have already mentioned that what we see reflects feelings more than what we hear. As students of kinesics, we should enhance our use of body language to reinforce our messages. We must strive to improve our ability to detect and interpret visual signals from others.

When we say one thing with words and something entirely different with facial expressions or voice tone ("mixed message"), we confuse our listeners.

Many facial expressions and gestures are familiar even to young children. Smiles, scowls, fist shaking, and "the high five" are easy to decipher. However, "steepling" (placing the hands in a prayerlike position), turning the palms down, or nose touching are signs that may be overlooked or misinterpreted.

Lack of eye contact may indicate insecurity, boredom or dishonesty. Some cultures forbid eye keying, regarding it as a sign of impoliteness or disrespect. Skilled interviewers and salespersons maintain eye-to-face contact without staring down the other person. Also, eyelids themselves deliver messages. When a person looks straight up at the ceiling while blinking rapidly, he may be exasperated, or may have already made up his mind. When he looks upward and to the left or right, it usually means that he is attentive or interested. One raised eyebrow indicates disbelief; when they both go up it is a sign of surprise.

Body position is important. Try to maintain the same eye level with the other person. Every parent knows that communication with tots improves when the parent gets down on the floor with the little ones. When talking to a bedridden patient, sit in a chair next to the bed. Sit upright and lean forward to show interest. Maintain a column of air between your back and the back of the chair.

On the other hand, if you want to inject more power into something you are saying at a meeting, stand up as you talk.

Head tilting may indicate acceptance, vulnerability, or comfort, or be an encouragement to more contact. Shortening the neck by raising shoulders is a subconscious protective move.

Touching is a sensitive issue. One must differentiate between social and business touching. Social friendships would be impersonal without an occasional hug or long handclasp, but these are inappropriate at work. The recent emphasis on sexual harassment has led some advisors to recommend against all body contact. That is unfortunate. Touching is a powerful communication tool if not abused. Important touch features are location, kind, and context.

Touches should be limited to handshakes (without lengthy holding), and light touches to the back of the forearm. Patting or massaging is verboten. Pats are bad because they may be interpreted as sexually oriented or patronizing (like petting a dog).

The touch should reinforce the verbal message. It is especially appropriate when expressing appreciation or support. Touches on the back of the forearm show emphasis when the toucher is talking, empathy when listening.

Customers are not exempted from the touching rules. Assertive recipients of unwanted contacts should say exactly how they feel about such liberties: "I know you don't mean anything by it, but when you put your arm around me it makes me uncomfortable."

It has been said that our feet are under least conscious control. A circular foot motion usually signals impatience. When a shoe hangs loosely on the forefoot, the person almost certainly is relaxed.

But be cautious about interpreting subtle visual messages. Do not rely on only one or two signs. A person may rub her nose because it itches. A person may cover his mouth because he had onions for lunch. Always look for confirmation in the form of other signs.

Signs of Attentiveness or Interest

When a person leans forward, smiles, and nods, he likes what he hears. Other signs of interest or agreement are manifested when he:

rubs his chin.
places his arms in front on the table.
sits erect.
rolls his eyes up and to the left or right.
maintains eye contact.
touches the other person.
holds his palms up.

Signs of Impatience

Be very sensitive to these when dealing with clients. If you are sitting in a client's office and she starts avoiding eye contact, looking at her watch, shuffling papers, playing with a paperclip, or placing her hand on the telephone, you have overstayed your welcome. If she stands up and starts to walk around her desk toward the door, you have been an insensitive clod.

Signs of Disinterest or Disagreement

If you are trying to make a point and your listener frowns, shakes his head, raises one eyebrow, and drums his fingers, your proposal is in big trouble. Other signs of disinterest, disbelief, or disagreement are:

eyes rolled up straight.
hand over mouth.
nose touching or rubbing.
head down, eyes straight ahead.
arms folded across chest.
leaning back or slouching down.
tugging on ear.
shoulders hunched.

Signs of Concealment or Nervousness

Many people believe that deception is revealed through the eyes or the face. Some research, however, suggests that signs of lying are better observed through body movement.[4] Admittedly, it is difficult to differentiate between nervousness and deceitfulness. One helpful discriminator is the articulation of a lot of "to tell the truths" or "honestlys." Your skepticism should vary directly with the number of these you hear. Here are some other helpful signals of untruthfulness.

squirming or fidgeting.
fast-blinking eyelids.
touching of mouth or nose.
back of hand up or toward listener.
evasive eye contact.
hand over mouth or eyes.
nervous fingers or feet.

Signs of Honesty or Openness

Head tilted to one side.
Open coat.
Palms up or toward listener.
Arms outstretched with palms forward.
Constant eye contact.

Signs of Confidence or Power

Many gestures signify power, some much more than others. These include:

clasping hands behind the head.
raising eye level (standing over person, sitting on edge of desk).
peering over the top of reading glasses.
"steepling."
placing hands on hips.
finger pointing and fist making.
extending head forward with lips drawn, frowning.
taking up more space, eg, resting arm on next chair, spreading out legs, placing
   briefcase on other person's desk.

Powerlessness is evidenced by using minimal body space, keeping feet crossed and hands folded on the lap. The message is "don't pay attention to me, I'm not important." Sitting stiffly with feet close together and arms close to side gives the true signal, "scared stiff."

Another Kind of Sign Language

How about our workplace signs? Are they positive or negative? Do they say what the clients or visitors can do or what they can't do? Are they helpful or inhibiting? Do most start or end with "Not permitted," "Don't," or "No?"

REFERENCES

1. Werther WB Jr: *Dear Boss.* New York, Meadowbrook Press, 1989.

2. Walther GR: *Phone Power.* New York, GP Putnam's Sons, 1986.

3. Bandler R, Grinder J: *Frogs Into Princes: Neurolinguistic Programming.* Moab, Utah, Real People Press, 1979.

4. Henderson PE: Communication without words. *Personnel J* 1989;68:22–32.

12. Use and Abuse of the Telephone

THE RINGING TELEPHONE heralds the start of a customer relationship.[1] How your telephone is answered says a lot about you and your department. An answering voice may express an affirmative, helpful attitude or an "I don't really care" one.[2]

While laboratories have relatively few person-to-person contacts with external clients, the number of telephone contacts with customers is usually great. Complaints about the amount of time spent in group meetings abound, but scheduled meetings account for one third less time than phone calls.[3] Lines tied up on personal calls can anger callers and cost money, and being transferred from one unit to another and then another is frustrating. When one of your clients hangs up, what do you think she says about you and your unit?

The same considerate, well-mannered, friendly people we know become ill-mannered, abrupt, and inconsiderate on the telephone.[4] Our telephone is so taken for granted that we hardly pause to question whether there is a way we could use it more effectively. All of us can use some brushing up.

ADVANTAGES OF INSTITUTIONAL TRAINING PROGRAMS

Everyone assumes that he or she knows how to use the telephone. Therefore, it is embarrassing, even insulting, to suggest to Louise that she should go off and take a workshop in telephone courtesy. This sensitive issue can be avoided if the organization offers periodic training programs for the entire staff, or management includes this training in its orientation protocol. An added benefit is that such group education promotes uniform telephone etiquette, which in turn has a reinforcing effect.

There are excellent workshops, professional speakers, and books available. Your telephone company can supply booklets and pamphlets that contain helpful suggestions for handling all types of calls.

VOICE QUALITY

You dial a number. The answering voice is warm and pleasant, welcoming the call. Diction is clear, the words easy to understand. Your first impression of that organization is very favorable.

We say that a voice has good quality or tone. Voice tone is actually the sum of speaking rate, volume, pitch, inflections, and choice of words. It is the varying of these factors that avoids the synthesized voice sound of robots.

Hire receptionists who speak impeccable English and have a pleasing voice tone. People spend hours listening to home audio systems before they purchase one. Managers should be just as choosy when hiring a telephone operator.

It is up to you to decide how your staff uses the telephone. Sit down with your secretary and develop a protocol for telephone usage. Cover everything from the way you want the telephone answered and calls transferred, to how to handle irate or disgruntled clients.[4]

How to Answer the Telephone

1. Identify yourself.
2. Identify the organization or department.
3. Offer to help.

Try to answer calls on the first or second ring. Quick responses reflect efficiency. Apologize if more than three rings were necessary. Answer with a friendly, smiling greeting. Yes, smiles are transmitted over telephone wires. For example:

"Good morning. Clinical laboratory. May I help you?" (Articulate the "morning" at a higher pitch to inject enthusiasm. Say it to yourself right now and see.)

"Good morning. Laboratory office. Linda speaking. How may I help you?" (Avoid using nicknames.)

"Clinical Laboratory." (This may suffice, especially when calls come in very quickly. It's better to shorten the salutation than to deliver a longer, rapid-fire, unintelligible greeting.)

FIVE WAYS TO AVOID TELEPHONE TAG

We all have experienced the frustration of failing to complete a call, and then being unavailable when the calls are returned. This can go on for hours, even days, and can also be expensive when the calls are long distance ones.

1. Pick the best time to call. People are most likely to be in their offices just before lunch and late in the afternoon. Ask the people being called, or ask their secretaries, for the best time to call, and write it down. Say when you will call again. Ask to have that information placed on the person's desk.
2. Ask to have person paged, or ask if there is another number at which person can be reached.
3. Ask if there is someone else who can answer your question.
4. Leave a message.
5. Use an answering machine, or the more sophisticated "voice mail" systems now available for personal computers.

Screening Calls

If it is necessary to screen calls, do it politely and tactfully. Screening usually provokes disappointment, often hostility, on the part of the caller. An effective screener helps callers by trying to answer their questions or by directing them to someone else who can answer them. To avoid transfers to wrong parties, the screener must be knowledgeable about departmental matters.

People who screen your calls should know which callers are always to be put through immediately, and those you never want to talk to. They should know what kinds of questions or problems you want to handle personally, and which ones can be referred, and to whom. Define emergency and urgent calls, and calls that can be classified as not urgent or nuisances. Screeners should make special efforts to get the important call to you.

The explosion of telemarketing has created a special problem. Most solicitations, whether for charitable organizations or business purposes, are insupportable. On the other hand, we do want to hear from certain sales reps and professional organizations. The increasing use of FAX machines for telemarketing poses a similar problem.

The phraseology used in screening calls is important. Here are some phrases that are overused, give the wrong impression, or are downright rude:

"Ms Smith hasn't come in yet."
"Joe just stepped out."
"She's in a meeting." (We don't believe this anymore.)
"He's in the john" (No kidding, I got that one from a "professional" employee.)
"You'll have to call back."
"We don't take these calls."
"You'll have to talk to me about that."
"What's your name and what do you want?"

Here is what you should hear:

"Dr Jones is out of his office right now, May I ask him to call you?"
"May I have your name, please?"
"He's not available at the moment; may I tell him who called?"
"Doctor, Miss Smith is meeting with our supervisors. The meeting usually ends

by 0900, may I have her call you then?"

"He's not in right now. I expect him back about 1400. Will you be available then?"

"Yes, she's in. May I tell her who's calling please?" (Do not ask for the caller's name before telling him or her that the person is not in.)

TRANSFERRING CALLS

Being transferred from one extension to another is a frequent source of irritation. Here are the four essentials of a courteous transfer:

The caller is given an explanation as to why he is being transferred.[2]

The caller is given the name, title, and extension number of the person to whom she is being transferred, so if she is disconnected she can reach that person with another call.[2]

Before the transfer is made, the secretary reassures the caller: "I'm sure that Ms Jones will be able to answer your questions."[2]

The secretary does not hang up until the connection has been made.[3]

PLACING ON HOLD

Apologize for not being able to connect the caller. Offer a choice of waiting or being called back. Check on the caller every 30 seconds while she is holding and repeat the offer. Background music does not substitute for courtesy. In fact, some callers are irritated by the music because they think it signals a longer wait.

If the caller says that she prefers to be called back, make sure that this is done.

TAKING MESSAGES

Walther[3] recommends getting rid of the "little pink slips" in favor of forms that have enough space for the following information:

1. name of caller. Phonetic version if the name is difficult to pronounce.
2. caller's organization or department.
3. caller's telephone number.
4. time and date of call.
5. purpose of call.
6. interpretation of caller's mood if he or she sounds upset, angry, or euphoric.
7. promises made to caller.
8. caller's unwillingness to talk to anyone else.
9. any previous important contacts with caller. It may be appropriate to attach copies of previous correspondence.

YOUR OWN TELEPHONE MANNERS

Who should take precedence, a visitor or a telephone caller? How would you feel if you were being interviewed for a job, and the interviewer accepted a longwinded call from a salesperson? That would tell you how you rate, wouldn't it?

When you have a visitor in your office, do not take calls unless they are urgent. If you are on the phone when a visitor who has an appointment arrives, quickly complete the call, or tell the person on the line that you will call back. If you are in someone else's office and an urgent telephone call for her interrupts, offer to step outside.[2]

If you have to cut the call short, explain why. Think about your diction and voice quality. Keep the conversation brief and to the point. If you want to terminate a rambling monologue, interrupt with something like: "Alice, I've got a meeting in one minute," (this does not have to be a lie—you can meet with yourself) or "Alice, I'm expecting an important call." (Aren't we always?)

ENDING CALLS

In telephone conversations, as in interviews or written correspondence, the beginnings and the endings make the strongest impressions. Conclude calls with a verification of key points covered.[3]

You want to be remembered as a pleasant, efficient person to deal with. Therefore, take the time to thank the person for calling, and say you were glad to be of service (or sorry that you couldn't help).

End the conversation on a pleasant upbeat note, but refrain from using that tiresome cliche "Have a nice day" or, even worse, "bye-bye." Instead say "It was nice hearing from you again," or "Thank you for filling me in—I appreciate it." If you know the person's family, you may refer to them before hanging up: "Give Sue and the kids my best."[2] Let the caller hang up first.

OUTBOUND CALLS

Have an up-to-date telephone directory close at hand. Keep a list of frequently called persons and their telephone numbers, the best time to call, and any other helpful information, such as their wives' names.

Set aside a time each day during which to make outbound calls. Avoid calls before 0900, after 1700, or between 1200 and 1330 hours. Most people do not like to be called at home when the subject is one that can be handled during the workday. Keep in mind any time differences when you make long-distance calls.

Plan ahead what you are going to say. Always retrieve any documents you might need.

Let the telephone ring eight to ten times before hanging up. If your secretary initiates the calls, make certain that you remain close by. It is irritating to the person being contacted and embarrassing to your secretary when you have to be hunted for.

Start conversations by stating your name; do not wait to be asked. If you are not well acquainted with the person you are calling, ask the switchboard operator how the person's name is pronounced, the name of her secretary, and her extension number in case the first call does not get through.

Ten Ways to Power up Your Language

1. Get your mind off other work; concentrate on that call.
2. Adjust your speaking rate and voice volume to that of the other person.
3. Get to the point quickly, and be brief. The suggestion has been made that longwinded people place an egg timer next to the phone to use as a reminder to keep calls short.[4]
4. Let the other person speak without interrupting.
5. Do not remain completely silent. This is disconcerting to the other person. Respond with "I see . . . Uh-huh . . . Interesting . . . Tell me more . . . Go on . . . Then what happened."
6. Develop rapport by using the person's name frequently, and asking for his and her viewpoint.[3]
7. Take notes.
8. Repeat and verify facts.
9. Save small talk for last.
10. Use the right words.
    Say what you *can* do, not what you can't.
    Avoid words that irritate, like "our policy" or "you'll have to."
    Avoid weasel words like "maybe" or "I'll try."
    In your statements, avoid cliches, fillers, and words that evoke hostility. Fillers are words like "Ya know."
    Use "I" language instead of "You" language: "You must be mistaken." (bad) "I think there may be a misunderstanding." (good)
    Say "no" without feeling guilty. Soften with "I wish I could help," or "I'm not free to release that information."
    Interrupt without being rude.

IMPORTANCE OF BODY LANGUAGE

A disadvantage of telephone communication is that it eliminates body language. But does it? True, the facial expressions, body positions, and gestures are not seen. However, researchers have shown that voices can often reveal when callers are smiling, sitting erect, or fidgeting in their chairs. These voice differences may be barely discernible to the conscious ear, but the subconscious mind "hears" them.[3]

Because some indicators of body language are transmitted during telephone conversations, act as you would if the person were sitting across from you. Sit erect. Use the same gestures. Smile so the person "sees" you smiling. Put a cartoon or a small mirror next to the telephone.

HANDLING IRATE CALLERS

In Chapter 15 I will discuss the handling of complaints, and difficult people in general. However, it is appropriate at this point to make a few comments that relate specifically to telephone situations.

Walther[3] suggests the following sequence for handling complaints:

1. Prepare yourself. Assume an executive posture. Have paper and pencil available.
2. Listen and record very carefully.
3. Encourage person to talk more. Ask open-ended questions. Use person's name frequently.
4. Solve their problems as best you can:
   Ask them for their solutions
   Speak in positive terms
   Sell the solution
5. Confirm and close. Review the complaint and the solutions. Be explicit.
6. Follow through.

Here are some appropriate responses[2]:

"I'm sorry to hear that . . . I'd be pleased to hear any suggestions you can offer."
"That's a great idea! I'll bring it up at our next staff meeting."
"I'm glad you brought this to my attention. What else happened?"

Even if you cannot help an unhappy customer, merely asking and listening is beneficial. When someone is complaining bitterly, ask her politely to repeat what she is saying, but to do it more slowly so you do not miss any of it.

When the caller is screaming at you and using profanity, and is obviously out of control, try this: Remain silent. Eventually the screamer will pause. She will wonder if you are still on the line (she has probably been through this before and had people hang up on her). She will stop her tirade and ask if you are still there. Her voice will now drop down several octaves, and she will talk more slowly. Respond with "Yes, I'm here. Please go on."

If a caller is unreasonable, suggest that he talk to someone higher up in the organization, and that you will be happy to arrange for that person to call him in a few minutes. Use those few minutes to brief the executive on the situation.[2]

THE ANSWERING MACHINE

Many people hate talking to an answering machine. Many just won't. For those of you who refuse to respond to these machines, I urge you to give the gadgets a fair shake. It is like pumping your own gas—as the machines become more familiar, they become less irritating. In fact, answering machines have some advantages over human contacts.

1. They force you to be brief.
2. You do not get any negative feedback or long-winded conversations.
3. Misinterpretation is less likely since the person can listen to the message as often as he or she likes.
4. They are great for reducing telephone tag.
5. If you do not want to be interrupted during interviews or other critical times, the answering machine can be as effective as a secretary.

Before recording your voice on your private machine, practice what you are going to say. A script can help. Listen to playbacks and keep recording your greeting until it is pleasant to listen to, and you sound enthusiastic. Baldrige recommends the following office message[2]:

"This is Ann Swift. When you hear the signal please leave your name, organization, and telephone number. I'll return your call as soon as possible. Thank you for calling."

Still better, invite the caller to leave a brief message. If the machine is at home, and you are frequently away for days at a time, ask the callers to state the day and time of their calls (some machines do this automatically).

REFERENCES

1. Goldzimer LS: *'I'm First': Your Customer's Message to You*. New York, Rawson Associates, 1989.
2. Baldrige L: *Letitia Baldrige's Complete Guide to Executive Manners*. New York, Rawson Associates, 1985.
3. Walther GR: *Phone Power*. New York, GP Putnam's Sons, 1986.
4. The use and abuse of the telephone. *Supervisory Sense* 1981;2:2.

(Note: All references were carefully selected and are worthy of additional reading. The book by Walther[3] belongs on your bookshelf. Read and reread it. Loan it out to your teammates. It is only a little book, but it contains a wealth of practical material.)

13. Written Communications

O N A DAILY basis, managers select channels of communication when contacting customers, including their employee-customers. Every year, the menu of choices expands, and these selections affect efficiency, expense, and client satisfaction.

When communication is verbal, should it be:

one-on-one? in my office, her office or elsewhere? a group meeting? via intercom? by word-of-mouth? a teleconference?

If communication is written, should it be a:

memo? letter? telegram? facsimile (FAX)? computer message?

Verbal communication is usually faster, permits complex dialogues, and transmits feelings better. Written messages can mute hostility or emotion, are permanent, and usually (but not always) are less susceptible to misinterpretation. Booher[1] recommends verbal communications (1) when you want immediate feedback, (2) when you want to persuade or question, and (3) when you do not want your words to come back to haunt you.[1]

Written messages do not interrupt their recipients like verbal messages frequently do. Busy people are annoyed by telephone interruptions or a summons to unscheduled meetings.

Written messages are usually more expensive. In 1985 a simple two-line typed letter dictated to a machine cost $6.22. When dictated fact-to-face the cost was $8.52, and even more if written by hand.[1]

A conversation should be followed by a memo or letter when:

a permanent record is needed.

the receiver is a poor listener, or is forgetful.

the oral communication may have been flawed.

more details are needed.

no action followed a verbal request.

senders want to make certain that they get credit for an idea.

(Note: Do not use memos to deliver bad news such as a firing, reprimand, or unpleasant assignment. Deliver these in person.)

CLIENT CONSIDERATION

Most managers and customers prefer one form of communication over the other. Obviously it pays to know which your boss and each of your clients like more, eg, many clients refuse to leave messages on answering machines. Customer satisfaction goes beyond selecting the preferred communication modality. It is more than a lot of "thank yous," "pleases" and stroking words. It is being tactful and considerate. It is taking into consideration the client's level of education and knowledge. It is making it easy for the client to respond, and not wasting his or her time by sending confusing messages.

LETTER *V* MEMO

Letters are for external communication, private, internal communication, or formal invitations. Memos, "messages in shirt-sleeves," are preferred for in-house, nonprivate messages. Figure 13.1 shows a recommended format for memoranda.

THE ABC RULE FOR GETTING ACTION

*A*ttention. You must get it.

*B*ehavior. What do you want the reader to do or what are you going to do?

*C*onvince. Provide facts, logic, statistics, or references.

THE THREE KEY STEPS IN WRITING LETTERS, MEMOS, OR REPORTS

1. Write a rough draft
2. Rewrite
3. Edit

1. Write a Rough Draft

Strive for a high-impact style to reduce reading time, provide better message comprehension, and eliminate the need for rereading.

To:	Night supervisor
From:	Lab manager
Date:	8/1/90
Subject:	New procedure for . . .
Message:	The new procedure will be demonstrated on 8/15/90 in the chemistry lab.
Action:	Please review the attached . . . and please attend the demonstration.
Attachments:	Procedure sheet for . . . .
Signature:	Sue Smith, Lab Manager
Copies to:	Medical director/Chemistry supervisor

Figure 13.1 A standard format for memos.

Write in a conversational mode. Imagine the reader sitting across from you. Start off with the person's name or with a "you." Try to deliver some good news, a compliment, or an expression of appreciation for something the person said or did.

Use a verbal hook to stimulate the reader's interest ("You're going to like what we're doing about your recent suggestion"). Include in the opening paragraph the purpose of the report and a summary sentence. Remember the newspapers' law of primacy: the first paragraph gets the most attention. Then prepare a strong closing statement. Accordng to the law of recency, the last paragraph gets the next most attention. Do not waste time by correcting grammatical errors or spelling in the first draft. Concern yourself only with content and clarity at this point.

2. Rewrite

Check the rough draft for brevity, clarity, and personal touch. Does it answer what, who, when, where, why, and how? Improve the readability as follows:

Use stroking words: the reader's name, "you," and "we," and compliments and expressions of appreciation.

Convert negative or impolite statements into positive, tactful, and courteous ones:

"You get late reports because your requests are usually late." (bad)
"When we get requests before 0700, our reports are rarely late." (better)
Note that the accusatory "you" is eliminated, and the focus is on the activity and solution.

Strengthen vague or abstract wording:

"We're going to decrease the turnaround time appreciably." (poor)
"We will cut turnaround time by one hour." (more precise)

chairman	chair, chairperson
foreman	supervisor
repairman	repairer
man-hours	work hours, staff hours
mankind	humanity
man the office	staff the office
Dear Sir:	Dear Friend (Customer, Colleague)

Figure 13.2   Revision of masculine names.[2]

Use gender-inclusive language. If you want to incur the wrath of women, use only male pronouns. Stereotyping women as secretaries and men as managers is even worse. While it is not possible to eliminate "man" from all words (penmanship, manager, mankind), most words can be desexed. Examples are shown in Figure 13.2.

The simplest way to neuter sentences is to use "he or she," but this gets cumbersome. Substitute titles, such as "the employee." In this book you may have noticed that I often balance the sexes by using "he" in one paragraph or sentence, and "she" in the next, always being careful not to stereotype male managers and female clerks.

3. Edit Carefully

Check the paragraphs. Keep them short, with one major thought for each.
Check the sentences. Vary their lengths to avoid a telegraphic sound. Break up the long ones.
Convert passive to active voice:

"Our monthly meeting has been discontinued." (passive)
"I have decided to discontinue monthly meetings." (active) (*Note:* The passive tense is sometimes better for diplomatic reasons.[2] It softens statements and avoids finger pointing:
"Credit cannot be extended to you at this time."
"An objection to your appointment was raised.")

Convert *-ion* nouns into verbs:
"It is my intention." ("I intend.")

Eliminate several kinds of words:

archaic, pompous, or overused phrases, and jargon like "bizlish," and "legalese" (Figure 13.3).
unnecessary words—"parasites," and "deadbeats."
"The consensus *of opinion.*"

Inform us as to your preference. (Which would you like?)

Upon receipt of your reply. (When we hear from you.)

Please advise us. (Please tell us.)

Pursuant to your request. (As you asked.)

If I can render. (If I can give.)

Permit me to explain. (Omit. Go ahead and explain.)

Please be advised. (Skip.)

I remain yours truly. (Yours truly.)

Figure 13.3   Avoid these "bizlish" and "legalese" phrases.

"It is a gray *color* and has a round *shape*."
redundant phrases or modifiers (Figure 13.4).
"there are" or "there is."
   "There are too many people arriving late."
   ("Too many people arrive late.")
weak words. Substitute strong ones.
   "We provide good service." ("We give outstanding service.")
excess pronouns and prepositions.
   "The decrease in profit is of great concern to us."
   ("We're concerned about decreased profit.")
slang, jargon, or acronyms.
buzzwords or hackneyed phrases like "interface," "down the tubes," "out of this
   world," "viable," "belly-up," and "bottom line."

Avoid contractions, such as "you're," except in personal correspondence.

Emphasize by underlining, highlighting, and using bold or italic print.

Check punctuation and spelling. The latter has been facilitated by the spell-
   checking software now available for most personal computers.

GENERAL SUGGESTIONS

How to Edit a Staff Member's Paper Inoffensively

Do not send it back to him all marked up like a school paper. Go over it in person.
Have him sit next to you while he holds his paper.

   Focus on major defects. Is the piece organized logically? Are statements
supported by data? Does it clearly state its purpose? Give specific examples of
what is still needed.

   Avoid finding too many flaws. The writer will think you are nitpicking. End
with an encouraging comment about how his reports have improved in content,
readability, or promptness.

Redundant Expressions	Preferred
Actual experience	Experience
Advance warning	Warning
Arrive on the scene	Arrive
Completely destroyed	Destroyed
Consensus of opinion	Consensus
Few in number	Few
Filled to capacity	Filled
Join together	Join
Just recently	Recently
My personal opinion	I think
Past experience	Experience
Postponed until later	Postponed
In view of the fact	Since

Figure 13.4 Redundant expressions.

How to Address Specific Situations

Problem Solving Letter

It is often necessary to respond to a customer's complaint or a request to resolve a service problem. The PAS approach of Brill[3] is recommended.

Problem: "Discourteous receptionist"
Analysis: "On-site observations by supervisor confirm complaint."
Solution: "The receptionist has been reassigned to clerical duties."

The "Sandwich" Technique for Saying "No" Diplomatically

Start off with something positive:
    "Your suggestion has obvious merit."
Deliver the bad news:
    "Budgetary restrictions prevent us from acting."
Say something positive:
    "We appreciate your interest and look forward to more of your good ideas."

How to Write a Commendation

Oral and written commendations represent praise in its highest form. Some managers are very stingy with praise. Others give verbal praise freely but seldom reinforce it with written commendations. In some instances this is because the manager doesn't know how to document the citation. These dos and don'ts are offered by Booher[1]:

State the overall commendation.
Be specific.
Be informal. Think of the memo as a warm handshake.
Name names when commending a group.
Be modest. Don't claim credit for yourself.
Do not focus only on benefits to the organization. Also mention how it benefits the
    person receiving the praise.

How to Document a Mild Reprimand

Passive-voice construction and "I" language are useful in preserving self-esteem: "The next time this situation arises, here is how I want it handled, Sue."

Turn your attention to the remedial steps taken by you or by others. Suggest how to avoid the difficulty in the future.

Do not understate or exaggerate the seriousness of the situation. Do not assume that the error was intentional or due to carelessness. Be willing to accept part of the blame. Do not attack character, personality, or work ethic. Do not patronize or be sarcastic.

How to Express Regrets Over an Error

Report the error promptly, and state how it was corrected. Provide a brief explanation and apologize. Take full responsibility for the mistake. Passing the buck only diminishes others' respect for you.

Do not overdo the apology. Overblown apologies and explanations sound insincere. Do not promise that the mistake will never occur in the future; but do explain what you have done to minimize that possibility. [1]

REFERENCES

1. Booher D: *Send Me a Memo: A Handbook of Model Memos.* New York, Facts on File Inc, 1984.
2. Baugh LS, Fryar M, Thomas D: *Handbook for Business Writing.* Lincolnwood, Ill, NTC Business Books, 1986.
3. Brill L: *Business Writing Quick and Easy.* New York, AMACOM Book Division, 1981.

14. Introducing Change

IN THE WORLD we work in, nothing is as constant as change. There are significant differences between the ways successful and not so successful organizations cope with changes. The winners are change specialists. They view changes as opportunities, and they know that to win they must be flexible and must be able to respond faster than their competitors.

In business, competition often follows a predictable chronologic sequence. A brand-new service provides an edge: "We have it, they don't." When rivals catch up, the advantage goes to the one with better quality: "We give you a lifetime guarantee." Later, the purchase price may have to be lowered: "We will not be undersold." When these three factors even out, the sales pitch focuses on customer service: "Our customers are always right." In each of these four competitive stances, change is involved—sometimes drastic—affecting everyone in an organization. An inability to react effectively may spell insolvency.

The first three competitive advantages (new service, quality, and price) are "high-tech," the fourth (customer service) is "high-touch," which refers to the person-to-person contact between customer and service provider. Laboratory improvements are usually of the high-tech variety, dealing with instrumentation, new services, quality assurance, management information systems, or work flows. High-touch improvements get less attention, but are obviously no less important, and, besides, they are free.

GETTING READY FOR CHANGE

A well-defined goal is a prerequisite for productive action, and embraces four critical objectives: (1) Selecting the right people; (2) Preparing and motivating people to change; (3) Obtaining the other necessary resources; (4) Implementing the change.

Plans and Strategy

The senior staff provides overall strategy and broad directives. It translates visions into concrete strategies. Middle- or first-level managers convert strategies into practical objectives, mobilize resources, and activate the changes.[1]

Every successful change starts with a workable, clearly defined master plan that is committed to writing. The plan answers the following crucial "W" questions:

What are our goals and objectives? What will it cost? What will we achieve? What environmental factors such as lighting and furniture must be considered? What are the risks, constraints, and barriers? What additional data are needed? What resources are essential? What did we do wrong last time?

Who wants the change? Why? Who benefits? Who will be affected adversely? Who will resist? Who will support us?

When should planning start? When will we have the time? When must we have approval? When should it be in operation?

Where do we start? Where will we find the space, funds, and people?

Will the change provide an opportunity to utilize available skills better? Will people have more autonomy over how they do their work? Will the changes make employees' jobs (and yours) easier or harder? Will the change increase or decrease profit (or motivation, morale, quality, or productivity)?

(**A caveat:** All successful plans are revised many times over the course of implementation.[1])

Gather Information About Previous Successes and Failures

Success Breeds Success.

The best predictor of future success is a history of previous successes. Experience is still our best teacher. Focus on activities that were instrumental in achieving success and those that were barriers to it. Evaluate your last change using the checklist in Figure 14.1. Assess the compatibility of the proposed change with the current organizational values and goals.

Design incentive and reward systems into the plan. Consider training to help prepare affected employees. Try to inject opportunities to eliminate tedious tasks, upgrade job skills, and increase flexibility. Consider contingencies for displaced people.[2]

Test your plan by asking these questions:

1. Is it concise and clearly written? Does it include action steps?
2. Was it distributed to the right people?
3. Has there been sufficient input from others?
4. Is there both a formal and informal network to lend credence and support?[1]

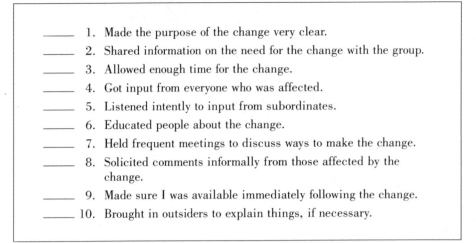

_____ 1. Made the purpose of the change very clear.

_____ 2. Shared information on the need for the change with the group.

_____ 3. Allowed enough time for the change.

_____ 4. Got input from everyone who was affected.

_____ 5. Listened intently to input from subordinates.

_____ 6. Educated people about the change.

_____ 7. Held frequent meetings to discuss ways to make the change.

_____ 8. Solicited comments informally from those affected by the change.

_____ 9. Made sure I was available immediately following the change.

_____ 10. Brought in outsiders to explain things, if necessary.

Figure 14.1   Evaluate your change efforts with this checklist. Consider the last change you made within your group. Check off those items on the list that you feel you handled satisfactorily.

WRITING A PROPOSAL

A proposal is actually a sales presentation.[3] As in all sales pitches, the more effective the presentation, the greater the chance for approval. The amount of justification required generally increases in proportion to the cost of a requested item.[4]

A creative proposal will get attention faster, so make it interesting and easy to read. A well-written proposal may not be approved, but it will win recognition and respect.[5]

How to Write a Proposal

Select an appropriate format. Many organizations have a standard form for proposals. If so, it simplifies organizing and outlining your document. A popular format is shown in Figure 14.2. For simple purchases of inexpensive items, a typed purchase order accompanied by a list of technical specifications and a vendor's quotation may be all that is needed.

The document should be easy to read. Box in special segments. Use headings, numbers, and indentations to divide the text. Allow plenty of white space (wide margins, double-spaced, space at top and bottom). Use high-quality paper and a letter-quality or laser printer. You want the document to look good but not ostentatious.

Make the report as factual as possible. When the data are "soft" or represent assumptions or personal opinions, say so.

Suggest how the proposal can be implemented and what possible difficulties may be encountered. Provide references and published information. Include alternatives and reasons for your selection. A good proposal will:

```
        I.  Overview
       II.  Description of current situation
      III.  Explanation of recommendation
            Benefits
            Methodology and research
            Expected results
            Specific action steps
       IV.  Experience of others
        V.  Potential vendors
       VI.  Costs
      VII.  Implementation timetable
     VIII.  Long-term plans
       IX.  Summary
```

Figure 14.2   Format for writing a proposal.

1. Define the problem or situation. To establish your credibility, show clearly that you know what the problem or current situation is, and that your proposal will correct it.[3]
2. Include goals and objectives. Goals describe long-range benefits or general statements of purpose. Objectives incorporate problem- and time-specific behavioral criteria, for example:
   Goal: To improve telephone communication between transfusion service and users of blood components.
   Objectives: 1. Install additional telephone extension in blood bank.
             2. Equip transfusionists with pagers.
3. Summarize the plan. List key steps, major activities, personnel involved, and a timetable. Use workload records to justify the request.[4]
4. State how the customer or organization will benefit.
5. Include a projected budget showing anticipated revenue enhancement, cost savings, and customer service improvements. Include specific costs of labor, supplies, equipment, training, and remodeling, as well as other expenses.[5]
6. Justify the need for urgency of approval, eg, to take advantage of a vendor offer that has an expiration date.
7. Prepare a summary.[6] Include a statement that describes how you will evaluate the success of the venture.[3]
8. Select a format: memo, letter, or formal report. Most organizations provide special proposal forms and instructions. Some even provide skilled personnel to assist in the preparation of requests for grants.
9. Review the document. Read it from the recipient's viewpoint. Does it provide all the essentials and anticipate queries? Have all the terms been defined? Have you used abbreviations, acronymns, or buzzwords that may cause confusion?

Cover Letter

A cover page, or letter of transmittal, starts with the title and origin of the project, the title of the addressee, and the date. It then spells out in concise terms the contents of the attached report. For example:

"Attached is a proposal for . . . to be used in the . . . department. The cost of this instrument is . . . This instrument should save $ . . . each year and decrease the turnaround time by . . . %. We can save $ . . . if we order by . . ."

Appendices

Include as appendices documents that support your proposal.[5] Examples are listed below:

Summary of methods and analytical information.
Quantitative comparison of systems.
Detailed summary of costs, including depreciation costs.
Copy of vendors' proposals.
Technical specifications of proposed system.
Resumes, graphs, and references.[3,4]

Presentations

Important proposals usually must be supplemented by presentations to an executive team. In these instances, prepare special handouts and display charts. Practice to smooth out the presentations. The degree of professionalism exhibited has a great effect on the acceptance or rejection of the proposal. Incidentally, your proposal should not come as a surprise to those receiving it. Talk it up as much as you can beforehand. Serve as your own marketing agent.

Respect channels of authority. Your immediate superior should know and approve what you're up to, even though his or her approval is not mandatory.

KEY QUESTIONS IN INSTRUMENT SELECTION

In the clinical laboratory many, if not most, proposals are submitted for the purpose of obtaining instruments or other equipment. The chances for getting approval for the purchase or lease of these items is greatly enhanced if there is adequate documentation of the need for such an investment, and proof that the most appropriate instrument is recommended. Following are some key descriptors that should be addressed.

Cost   What is the total cost of the instrument, including putting it on line? Will the instrument really reduce costs? How much? Will maintenance costs be lower?

Time   Will it decrease turnaround time? When can it be installed? What downtime can be anticipated?

Quality   Will it improve quality?

1. Describe why a change is needed.
2. Relate its potential benefits.
3. Provide examples of how this has succeeded elsewhere.
4. Select the best time to present your case. Avoid discussing it during a crisis or a very busy period, such as just before an inspection.
5. If your boss seems detached or disinterested, say that you need more data. Come back another time.
6. Do not overstate your case. The moment your boss knows or even suspects that you are stretching the facts, he or she may discount your entire idea.
7. Do not try to gain acceptance by understating the costs or time involved.
8. Do not articulate your case apologetically.

Figure 14.3   How to recommend a change.

User Friendliness   Will it be easier to operate? Can it be used by all shifts? Can a less qualified person run it?

Special Requirements   Does it require additional space or facilities (power, ventilation and so forth)? Does it necessitate change in the work flow? What specimen volume is needed? Will supplies be readily available? Is it compatible with our computer? Must new forms be designed? (*Note:* Keep handy the emergency telephone numbers of vendors, experts, and other key people. In any large project you will need them.)

GARNERING SUPPORT

Sell the procedure to the power holders and the opinion leaders above and below you in the hierarchy. Ask people at all levels what the change is going to accomplish. Are their expectations similar?[1]

Support of top management is crucial. In many instances executives must provide more than the wherewithal. They must also participate actively in solving problems. Figure 14.3 lists suggestions on how to recommend a change.

Support From Your Employees

Let's say you have what you know is a good plan. You have researched it thoroughly, and have outlined the strategy. You have a tentative go-ahead from the top brass. Now you need the support of your staff. You wisely go for the "bottom-up" strategy, which is the best way to gain input and acceptance.

The Bottom-Up Strategy

The name of the game is PARTICIPATION. Ideally, this participation is introduced when change is first contemplated. Creating interest in something before it is a fait accompli helps to deflate resistance and lessen criticism.[7] The goal is to get the team to accept ownership, and the more input the group has, the greater its feeling of ownership.

Invite participation by everyone affected. Honor, respect, and reward creativity. Review available information and outline possible strategy and alternative methods for implementing the plans.[1] Use a variety of feedback tools, including responses to memos or inquiries. Share individual suggestions offered outside of scheduled group meetings. Widen your "open-door" policy. But if the plan is complete when presented to your team, don't pretend that modifications are still possible. This manipulation will be transparent.

IMPLEMENTING THE CHANGE

It is important not to fail at the start. Change masters arrange for a quick payoff by starting with the right group and a simple, limited action.[1]

The seven keys to successful implementation are as follows:

1. Clarify strategy and plans.
2. Mobilize resources. Choosing the right people is especially critical.
3. Introduce new practices slowly.
4. Provide needed education.
5. Give and get feedback continuously.
6. Run interference for the team members.
7. Don't nitpick or be a bottleneck.

If it is not possible for employees to participate in the planning sessions, it is even more important for them to be involved in designing the implementation process. When a team lacks ownership of a plan, getting commitment is more difficult. This commitment must be sincere. If you demand it, all you get is "lip service." Get public endorsement—it is more likely to last.

Participation in the implementation plans begins with the presentation of an easy-to-understand preliminary proposal that is subject to change after thorough discussion. The best-designed systems are effective only to the degree that people who man the systems understand and use them.

Use weekly meetings to discuss modifications and problems. Continue the group meetings throughout the implementation process. Define and emphasize common interests, taking into account the different viewpoints of various work groups and individuals. Interactions must include dialogues. Accept, even welcome, critical comments. A good sign is when the group talks about the change in "we" terms.[1] Empower employees to make changes happen. Build in incentives for using the change. Stay in touch with workers' daily efforts.

Try to get everyone involved. When a worker does not share a special relationship with other team members, he or she can become a marginal, noncontributing member—a spectator. And, like other spectators, this person will stand on the sidelines and heckle the players,[8] who have enough of a challenge without putting up with this kind of nonsense.

Maintain optimism and a sense of humor. Take set backs in stride. Do not let your frustration show. Your staffers take their cues from you.[9]

Good communication is a must. Communication is more than sending and receiving information. It is also being a cheerleader.

When associates report rumors, tell them as much as you can. Straight talk is essential to your credulity. Once associates know that they know what you know, they'll gain confidence.

TRAINING

"The best designed systems are effective only to the degree that the people who man the system understand and use them."[10]

Clarify training objectives through a thorough needs analysis. Ask the learners what they want, and incorporate their suggestions into the program. Design training that provides job-related skills. Enroll the highly motivated and influential users first.

Training sources include vendors, training consultants, and local experts who use a variety of educational techniques, and evaluate the effects of the training.

OVERCOMING RESISTANCE

"Almost always people individually and collectively resist the anxiety and uncertainty that change inevitably produces."[1] Resistance results in delays. Only in fables does the tortoise win. Resistance is loyalty to the past or present. Your aim is to switch loyalty from preserving daily work patterns to attaining new objectives of customer courtesy and responsiveness.[8]

Why do People Resist Change?

Some people thrive on change; most do not. The tolerance that people have for change is intimately connected to their motivational needs. Those whose principle motivational drive is toward power fear any change that reduces their influence. Those with strong social needs worry about their team being split up. Workers who get their satisfactions from task achievements view with suspicion any change that threatens their work routines.

Barriers to Change

The greatest barrier to change is fear.

1. General fear of the unknown. Changes force employees to face the unknown, whereas life before change was predictable and comfortable.[11]
2. Fear of failure. Most of our failures are at first attempts.
3. Economic fears:
   Loss of job.
   Demotion, transfer, or reassignment.
   Loss of overtime.

4. Personal fears.
   Too much work: "You expect us to do that and our job too?"
   Loss of territory or work space. People like a work space of 8 to 10 linear feet, and 4 to 6 linear feet of personal space.
   Loss of job satisfaction.
   No recognizable personal benefit.
   Perceived role change: less or more responsibility, less use of expertise.
   Overspecialization or loss of it.
   Implied criticism behind change.
   Dislike for learning new techniques.
5. Group fears.
   Change in working relationships.
   Lack of group participation.

   Other barriers include the following:

1. Satisfaction with the status quo. People like being on automatic pilot. Habits and patterns do not require much cerebration.
      "Things aren't really that bad."
      "If it ain't broke, don't fix it."
2. Inability to comprehend the need for change.
3. Previous negative experiences.
4. Unjustified pessimism with change:
   "Nothing we do will help."
   "They'll never let us do it our way."
   "Last year it was zero-based budgeting, what next?"
5. Vested interests.
6. Managerial deficiencies.
   Failure to consider the overall organizational goals and strategy.
   Failure to develop strategy and plans.
   Failure to recognize who will be affected, and to get their input and "ownership."
   Failure to mobilize the expertise needed.
   Failure to delegate.
   Ignoring barriers and complaints.
   Poor working relationship.

The first opposition to change may take place when news of possible change surfaces. This may come through the grapevine, or be transmitted by formal announcement at a staff meeting. Some employees sense that they will be affected but prefer to bury their heads in the sand. Others convince themselves that they will not be involved.

Group resistance often remains hidden until implementation takes place. Louise discovers that she must share her office with the laboratory information system (LIS) coordinator. Joe finds a new group around the coffee pot. A plan that looked so bright at first suddenly loses its luster.

If employee concerns are ignored, they escalate and are more difficult to alleviate.

Strategies for Dealing With Resistance

Participation

We have already discussed the importance of getting employees involved in planning and implementation. By involving people before specific changes are made, a leader confronts deep-seated, negative attitudes before they become barriers. People who participate and are empowered to control most of their activities become committed.

Education

Once workers realize that they will be retrained or reassigned their resistance often decreases. When employees are given instruction manuals, hands-on training, and the time to play around with new equipment, they quickly develop self-confidence.

People whose jobs are eliminated should have the benefit of outplacement services and career-planning programs.

Communication

The very act of talking about the change reduces fear and resistance, especially if you acknowledge concerns and anxieties as legitimate. Tell employees that what they feel is perfectly normal and that those feelings will pass.

"I'd rather fight than switch . . . back."

It helps to remember that once people have accepted and adjusted to change their attitude takes a 180° turn. Now they would fight against going back to the old method.[11]

Special Tips

Give people time to get used to the idea of a change.
Disagree without being disagreeable.
Be patient.
Avoid placing blame.
Admit mistakes.
Regard errors, yours and theirs, as learning experiences.
Do not aggravate or force defensiveness.
Use models and examples.

If past changes have ended in failure:

explain the change fully.
point out how this change is different.
start small and simple.
strive for success. If achieved, publicize it. [1]

Adjusting to Imposed Change

People may become ecstatic over changes they have originated. It takes a lot more effort to become enthusiastic over someone else's brainchild. If you are handed new responsibilities, new reporting requirements, or new people, find out how your daily routine will be affected. Project a cooperative attitude. Be supportive and enthusiastic. Serve as an influencer, rather than a reactor. Participate actively in the planning phase, and even become one of the experts or leaders.

Ask a lot of questions and do your homework. If change necessitates additional training or education, enroll in courses, seminars, and self-instruction programs dealing with your areas of responsibility.

If the change affects your staff, your procedures, or work in progress, initiate the necessary changes expeditiously. Seize on opportunities for yourself and members of your staff to enhance competencies, authority, or promotability. The change may invite territorial expansion or additional financial support. Do not neglect to take advantage of these opportunities.

How you cope with imposed change will be closely watched by your employees. You are their role model. If you drag your feet, do a lot of griping, and display a generally negative attitude, do not expect exemplary behavior on their part when you try to initiate one of your projects.

REFERENCES

1. Dalziel MM, Schoonover SC: *Changing Ways: A Practical Tool for Implementing Change Within Organizations*. New York, AMACOM Book Division, 1988.
2. Mainiero LA, DeMitchell RL: Minimizing employee resistance to technical change. *Personnel* 1986;63:32–37.
3. Knapp BO: Writing a proposal? No problem. *Training* 1988;25:55–57.
4. Werninghaus KA: A guide to writing winning proposals. *MLO* 1986;18:71–75.
5. Barros A: Writing effective proposals and job descriptions. *MLO* 1989;21:15–16.
6. West A, Anderson W: A polished proposal for laboratory funding. *MLO* 1985;17:79–82.
7. Harris TE: A partnership for change. *Manage World* 1989;3:15–16.

8. Gilbreath RD: The myths about winning over resistors to change. *Supervis Manage* 1990;35:1–3.

9. Kirby T: *The Can-Do Manager* New York, AMACOM Book Division, 1989.

10. O'Connell A: Making the new technology work. *Supervis Manage* 1990; 35:8–9.

11. Wickes TA: Techniques for managing change. In Preston P, Zimmer TW, eds: *Management for Supervisors.* Englewood Cliffs, NJ, Prentice-Hall, 1978.

15. Complaints and Complainers

O MATTER HOW unreasonable a complaint may seem to you, the client has the right to express it. No matter how unreasonable the client may seem to you, his complaint should be heard; it might be quite reasonable. All complaints must be given an open ear—regardless of the real validity of the problem.

The Three Kinds of Customers

1. The ones who are pleased with your service.
2. The ones who are displeased and tell you why.
3. The ones who are displeased, do not tell you, stop using your service, and tell everyone else.

Why Customers Complain

1. They did not receive what was promised or expected.
2. They had to wait.
3. Someone was rude, patronizing, aloof, disinterested, or unfriendly.
4. Someone gave them the runaround.
5. Someone ignored them, or did not listen.
6. Someone expressed a "can't do" attitude.
7. Someone hit them with the rulebook.

Why Customers Do Not
Complain More

Patients complain about food, prompt service, and courtesy, things they are qualified to rate. They are less apt to challenge professional competency. But this is changing as people gain more health-related knowledge.[1] Complaints from or concerning inpatients are usually more vehement because the hospital laboratory has a service monopoly. Lacking the choice available to outpatients, inpatients and their attending physicians have no recourse other than to complain.

Here are the principle reasons why people do not complain[2]:

They do not think it is worth the time and effort.
They do not think anything will be done about it.
They do not know where or how to complain.

Most customers are understanding, and stifle their irritation if they feel that providers care about them, understand their needs, and are doing their best to set things right.[2] However, this empathy dissipates rapidly if the server is rude, disinterested, or uncooperative.

HOW COMPANIES HANDLE COMPLAINTS

Most organizations have customer service departments, patients' representatives, or risk managers who investigate problems and promise to get back to the customer. They take the customer's version of what happened, get a different version from the employee, and may or may not send the customer a note offering an adjustment or an apology.

Client-oriented employers actively solicit complaints and let their customers adjust most of their grievances. At least they ask for the clients' opinions and make a special effort to make things right. They practice what they preach: "the customer is always right."

CHANNELS FOR REGISTERING COMPLAINTS

Complainers who tell us how to correct the situations constitute one of our most valuable problem-solving groups. In an earlier chapter we discussed the various means for obtaining customer feedback. At this point, let us concentrate on the complaint aspect. When you look for complaints, you are expressing interest, concern, and the desire to satisfy customers.[3]

Comment forms filled out by clients immediately after a service has been rendered are an inexpensive way to elicit current gripes. Mailed questionnaires are more expensive and the data are less current.

Incident reports and complaints should be recorded in a special file and reviewed frequently by an executive who regards them as a high-priority item and takes vigorous remedial action. Repetition of the same complaints points to a serious managerial deficiency.

All too often managers throw up their hands and blame customer dissatisfaction on employees who "have a poor work ethic." Who selected and indoctrinated those workers?

THE TEN STEPS IN DEALING WITH COMPLAINTS

1. Be approachable. Think of the last time you faced a physician, nurse, or patient who was complaining. What were your words, your voice tone, and your body language? Do you think the person perceived you as being patient and receptive, or annoyed and defensive?

What did you say the last time one of your associates brought you someone else's complaint? Did you start off with, "Not you again. Now what are they griping about?" or "Well, here comes Miss Bad News." Your poor response to these messengers of unpleasant tidings will determine how well you will be kept informed about your services. The complaints will still occur, but you will not know about them. When someone does bring up the subject, you can say with all sincerity, "Complaints? we must be doing OK, we don't get many complaints."

2. Hear the customer out without interrupting. Establish good rapport by responding appropriately. If the customer is friendly, be cheerful. If the customer is angry, show concern. If the customer is in a hurry, exhibit urgency. Use your very best active listening skill while remaining calm, interested, and attentive.

3. Make sure you understand the complaint. Ask as many questions as is necessary. This will not only clarify the situation, it will also indicate that you are interested in resolving the problem, and that you care.

4. Find something to agree on. Ask the customer what he or she wants done. This is a quick way to come up with a solution, and you may be surprised how little the person expects. It also prevents you from working toward the wrong solution.

5. Say what you can do, not what you cannot do. Avoid statements like "This department doesn't handle that," "that's impossible," or "that's not my responsibility." Accept the complainant's remedy or propose a solution and try to obtain his or her support. If the complainant does not like your solution, press for alternatives. If you cannot do what the complainant wants, do not say he or she is wrong. Explain why you cannot be accommodating.

6. If necessary, gently confront the complainant. Do not get into an argument. Do not be accusatory or challenging, eg, "You didn't get the request here on time." Instead, say: "The request arrived late." If the customer's tirade continues, use the "broken record" technique, repeating, "I'm sorry," or "I understand your concern."

If the customer threatens to go over your head, say, "That's your privilege, but I'd like to help you right now." If the complainant insists, or if you feel that you are unable to resolve the problem, transfer negotiations to your superior. Do it graciously.

7. Thank the customer. State that you always appreciate knowing about problems because it gives you an opportunity to correct the situation, and helps prevent similar problems in the future.[3] Invite the person to become a member of your network dealing with improving customer service.

8. Act. Implement corrective measures promptly, and do not just patch up the current situation. Do whatever is necessary to prevent a recurrence.

9. Inform the customer of your action. Say what you did and express the hope that he or she is satisfied and will continue to patronize your service. Ideally this

feedback should be as a telephone call from you, followed by a letter from your superior.

10. Record the complaint in your special log. You may also want to discuss the complaint and its resolution at your next staff meeting.

LISTENING SKILLS

Even if you cannot really help an unhappy customer, merely asking and listening helps. "Nothing deflates a fight-prone client faster than the chance to vent frustration to a nonargumentative, attentive listener."[4]

Keys to Active Listening

Active listening is nothing more than letting the other people know that you have heard and understood what they said. General principles of active listening were presented in Chapter 11, but some more specific suggestions are in order.

1. Know when not to talk. Silence is golden when it consists of pauses that encourage the other person to continue, and when it prevents you from saying what should not be said.
2. Show empathy by reflecting how the person feels. Use descriptive adjectives like upset, stressful, difficult, aggravating, or inconvenient.
3. Use "openers" to stimulate the dialogue, eg, "Tell me more," or "I'd like to know more about that."

Dos and Don'ts of Complaint Reception

Do concentrate on factual information.
Do give the person your complete attention.
Do show a caring attitude.
Do take notes if the complaint is lengthy.
Do use active listening.
Do use soothing words (Figure 15.1).
Do accept responsibility.
Do apologize.
Do end on a positive note.
Do take quick and effective action.
Do be specific as to what you're going to do and when.
Don't take complaints personally.
Don't react defensively.
Don't blame the computer.
Don't blame other people.
Don't minimize the complaint.
Don't use inflammatory words or phrases. They quickly make matters worse (Figure 15.2).
Don't make promises you can't keep.

"I'm sorry you had a problem with . . ."
"We're going to . . ."
"Thank you for giving me the chance to . . ."
"What do you think we should do?"
"That's a great idea. Thanks."
"Here's what we can do right now."
"As I understand it, you're upset because . . ."
"That is a problem. I don't blame you for complaining."
"I'm certainly glad that you saw me."
"You'd make a great troubleshooter."

Figure 15.1   Use these great phrases.

Don't make culpability statements that can get your organization in trouble, eg:
"Sorry about our lab error that led to the wrong diagnosis."

ANGER AND ANGRY CUSTOMERS

Anger is induced by embarrassment, disappointment, or frustration. It is much easier to cope with clients who are disappointed because you can reason with them. When angry people lose control, reasoning goes out the window. These people will not listen to explanations; they want action or someone's head.

Explanations seem logical, but not only are they usually a waste of time, they tend to irritate more. Only action convinces angry individuals that you are not trying to stonewall their grievances. Blaming computers, policies, or other people also fuels the fire. So does trying to shrug off responsibility, or claiming lack of authority to act.

Instead of shifting blame or providing excuses, ask the complainers for their solutions. This often stops them in their tracks. They usually have exploded before they thought the problem through to a solution.

Grant as much problem-solving authority as possible to the front-line troops. Complaints are resolved more quickly, and the service provider will like the increased responsibility and authority, increasing his or her self-esteem.

How to Diffuse Anger

Do not lose your cool. When you respond emotionally, you lose.
Listen, really listen. Do not interrupt.
Show, by words and body language, that what the complainant is saying is important. Say so!

disagree	have to	policy
no	must	can't
not my job	too busy	I only work here
rule	practice	It's the computer
unreasonable	tell them	understaffed
you're wrong	you serious?	I don't make the rules

Figure 15.2   Avoid these inflammatory words or phrases.

Deal with feelings first. Use nonjudgmental or empathetic phrases such as
  "appears as if," "seems as though" or "I can appreciate. . . ."
Use the client's name a lot.
Take notes. It shows that you care.
Make sure you know what the client wants.
Seek a win/win solution.
Act promptly.

THE HOSTILE COMPLAINERS

There are some special kinds of people whose anger or apparent anger is wrapped
in hostility.

The "Steamroller"

Steamrollers are those persons who always want to flatten you.[5] They are difficult
to handle because they usually have power, are very aggressive, and know exactly
what they want. Every medical staff has one or two of these (usually surgeons).
They can also be found in the executive suite.

   These folks act the way they do simply because it works almost all the time.
They do not hesitate to push to the head of a line, or to interrupt a meeting. They
act like they are angry, but it is just that—an act. Their emotions are under
complete control. These dictators bully, cajole, and intimidate. If you counterattack, there will be war. If you are passive, they destroy your confidence and self-
esteem.

Coping with Steamrollers

Instead of resisting, dodge. What happens in football when a huge lineman
lunges at a quarterback? The quarterback does not counterattack; he makes a
quick evasive move. The lineman not only misses, he usually falls down. One way
to move like a quarterback is to "go neutral."[6] To go neutral is to maintain control,
and not get angry. Silently and without expression you "look through" the person

as though he or she were not there.[6] This helps you to maintain eye contact and to maintain your poise without counterattacking.

Bramson's[5] aligning technique is more sophisticated. Here's how Bramson would have you deal with Dr Furious, a Steamroller:

1. Position is important. Maintain eye level and contact. Ask him to sit down. If he won't, you stand up.
2. Allow him to vent his feelings without interruption. When he runs out of breath, do not counterattack. Ask him to continue: "Dr Furious, I may disagree, but tell me more." Ask open-ended questions. Don't interrupt until he has had his complete say. Don't accuse him of anything. Don't complain or whine.
3. Respond forcefully. Insist that he listen to your response. He will probably interrupt you. Do not incur his wrath by saying "Stop interrupting me" or giving him a lecture on interrupting people. This only intensifies the conflict. Simply say, "Dr Furious, you interrupted me." Expect more interruptions, and respond the same way until he listens to what you have to say.
4. Switch to problem-solving. When he sees that he can't pulverize you, he will turn his attention to the problem that brought him there. Ask him for his suggestions.

The "Volcano"

The second group, called "exploders" by Bramson, consists of people who are ordinarily quiet and peaceful, but who periodically erupt like volcanos, spewing hot lava and sparks all over the place. Volcanos are really angry, and at least partially out of control.

The volcanos' tantrums are childlike and represent defensive reactions. In the past volcanos found that people did not take them seriously unless they threw a fit. Their attacks are usually precipitated by things that frustrate or embarrass them. They did not get what was promised, someone was rude, they were kept waiting, or they were the targets of kidding.

Coping With the Volcanos

Volcanos are handled somewhat differently than steamrollers. Since their anger is not under control and some of them strike, make allowance for a quick retreat. However, like windup toys, volcanos always run down if you can wait them out.

Try to get the person to sit down in a private area. If you fear physical abuse or she does not calm down, leave. Say "I can't listen when you use that tone of voice," or "I'll talk to you later."

When she pauses, say "Look, Mrs Jones, this is important. I want to hear every word, but not this way." Sound dramatic. Repeat if necessary. Use her name frequently. Ask her to repeat what she said but to talk slower. It is hard to talk angrily when you talk slowly.

Another approach is to say that you need a paper and pen to write down the facts. Go look for the paper. This gives her more time to wind down. Ask her to repeat what she just said. She will probably sit down and slow down. Get as much information as possible.

If an apology is in order, make it. But add that you do not like the way she is acting: "Mrs. Jones, I apologize for . . . but I don't like being called names or being yelled at. I can get your point without that." If she is still unsettled, suggest a later meeting.

After she has calmed down, she often will be embarrassed, even apologetic, and she may cry. At this point offer concrete help such as an investigation of the complaint or information or service for her. Say exactly what you are going to do and when: "Let me discuss this with my supervisor and get back to you. How about 9 AM tomorrow?" Be sure to get back to her.

The Profane Ones

Profanity is ingrained into some persons' conversation. Every sentence contains four-letter words. They mean no harm by this, and most of us can put up with it even though it is unpleasant.

There are those who turn on the foul language only when they are angry and out of control. None of us has to tolerate extreme profanity. All employees should have permission to walk away from such individuals, or to hang up the telephone after saying "Pardon me, I don't have to listen to this kind of language and I'm leaving [hanging up]."

EMPLOYEE COMPLAINTS

We must keep reminding ourselves that our associates are also our customers. As customers, they too are entitled to register complaints. Like other clients, many of their gripes concern treatment.

While it is obviously better to prevent complaints than to react to them, even the best-run organizations will receive some complaints from workers, including an occasional formal grievance. Complaint resolution is crucial to productivity and morale. Studies show that at unionized hospitals where complaints were resolved expeditiously and effectively, fewer strikes took place.

Causes of Employee Complaints

Employee complaints may result from employee-job mismatches, oppressive policies, an unpleasant working environment, perceived inadequate compensation or benefits, inept or unfair supervision, and conflicts with other employees or departments (Figure 15.3).

(Note: Most initial complaints are not the real ones; they are only trial balloons to see how bosses respond.)

A. The infrequent complainer with a valid complaint.
B. The chronic complainers
    1. People with personality or emotional disorders.
    2. Employees who hate their jobs, but cannot quit.
    3. Hostile, antiauthoritarian activists who resent taking orders.
    4. Emotional, unstable, or temperamental types who are easily wounded by any kind of criticism.

Figure 15.3 Classification of employee complainers.

Prevention of Complaints and Grievances

Most complaints and grievances can be prevented simply by eliminating the causes listed above. For starters, employers must abide by the limitations placed by collective bargaining agreements, antidiscrimination legislation, civil service regulations and employment contracts.

The more channels for expressing complaints, the better. Best are face-to-face meetings between the supervisor and the aggrieved person, and a delegate for the employee or a union representative. Many organizations have special counselors or committees to deal with employee problems. Open-door policies are highly recommended.

Gripes are often registered through suggestion boxes, notes or telephone calls (often anonymous), letters to newspapers, and notices from lawyers, the Occupational Safety and Health Agency, or the Equal Employment Opportunity Commission.

THE SUPERVISOR'S ROLE

1. Register the complaint by listening patiently. Remember that the complaint articulated may only be the tip of the iceberg or a smoke screen. Record the complaint in detail and to the satisfaction of the complainant. Ask what action the employee wants taken. Promise to look into the matter and to get back to the person.
2. Investigate by verifying what you have been told and determining if others have the same complaint. If appropriate, notify your superior or the human resources department.
3. Decide on your action. Use your problem-solving skill to consider alternatives. Ensure that your decision is compatible with company policies, governmental requirements and the union contract.
4. After making sure that you have the power to act, inform the employee of your proposed action. Try to do this within 24 hours. State exactly what is going to be done. If your solution is not acceptable, inform the person of his or her rights of appeal.
5. Implement the decision and get feedback on the effectiveness of your action.

HOW TO COPE WITH CHRONIC COMPLAINERS

Chronic complainers may be harmless, but some can damage morale and performance, and their constant griping can be contagious. They behave self-righteously and blame others. They are always in an accusatory mode. Their voices are plaintive, passive, and whining. Because they feel powerless, they make no effort to solve problems by themselves or in concert with others. Follow these steps when responding to chronic complainers:

1. Listen attentively, but only long enough to identify the problem. Stop the complainant as soon as you hear repetition.
2. Keep the chronic complainers busy. Complaints and other troubles surface when people are not constructively occupied or are underutilized. While activity is not a cure-all, it can remove some problems.
3. Acknowledge complaints and feelings, but do not agree (empathize, not sympathize). Make limiting responses such as, "You feel that you weren't treated well this week."
4. Ask probing questions such as: "When did you first notice that?" "Is it getting better or worse?" "What should be done?" "What have you done about it?" "How come you're the only one complaining?"
5. Take notes while listening. This will make the person feel that what he or she is saying is being taken seriously.
6. Take action if appropriate, but do not expect great results.
7. Insist that complaints not be voiced in front of patients, visitors, or other clients.

Four Big Don'ts

1. Don't agree that the complaints are correct, even if they are.
2. Don't try to placate, or explain everything.
3. Don't become defensive.
4. Don't apologize. You will only hear more complaints.

REFERENCES

1. Lochman JE: Factors related to patients' satisfaction and adherence associated with resident skill. *J Commun Health* 1983;9:91–109.
2. Walther GR: *Phone Power.* New York, GP Putnam's Sons, 1986.
3. Goldzimer, LS: *'I'm First': Your Customer's Message to You.* New York, Rawson Associates, 1989.
4. Oostra R, Young L: Six steps to deal with complaints about lab service. *MLO* 1988;20:65–70.
5. Bramson RM: *Coping with Difficult People.* New York, Anchor Books, 1981.
6. Mellot R: *Stress Management for Professionals.* Boulder, Colo, Career Track Publ, 1987.

16. Retention of Personnel

DAVIDOW AND UTTAL[1] put it very well when they wrote "The deadly enemy of great performance on the front line is high turnover. Nobody can be expected to shine when he's new on the job, doesn't know the technical aspects of his work or lacks the confidence to take risks on the customer's behalf." We have all experienced that sinking feeling we get when we're greeted with "Sorry, I'm new here."

Poor employee retention is expensive. The cost of replacing an employee may be equal to the annual salary of the vacated position. Employee retention is a growing problem in health care institutions because the need for professional and technical workers is increasing while the supply is shrinking. The annual turnover rate for most industries is about 12%,[2] while that for hospital nurses hovers around 30%.[3] In my own experience, that 30% probably applies to skilled laboratory workers as well.

The old response to personnel shortages was to step up recruitment, but administrators soon discovered that recruitment alone was only a quick fix. The focus then turned to retention strategies. Retaining employees is less expensive and less disruptive than replacing them.

WHY DO EMPLOYEES QUIT AND GO ELSEWHERE?

Chief executives prefer to believe that their employees are being enticed away. This absolves them of accountability for the departures, and begs a simple solution — more pay and benefits. Reasons for resigning are stated in letters of resignation, or in exit interviews. However, these data are flawed. Departing employees play it safe. Not wanting to jeopardize good references or the opportunity to return, they downplay dissatisfaction with the job and the people they are leaving.

First-line supervisors blame top management. They point to noncompetitive salaries, understaffing, objectionable work schedules, and other factors that they feel are out of their control. They do not realize that they, the supervisors, are often partly responsible for employee dissatisfaction. That is because few employees have the courage to confront their immediate superiors. Instead, they sublimate their feelings by directing their ire at top management. Zarandona and Camuso[4] challenged the validity of exit interviews. When they contacted resignees by telephone 18 months after the employees had resigned, they learned that almost 25% of them quit because of their immediate supervisor, twice as many as those who left for a better job.[4]

When employees say they do not receive recognition they are usually talking about their immediate boss. Most workers will stay on the job despite tremendous adversity as long as they feel that they are respected, can affect work with their ideas, and have a sense of belonging.[5]

How to Analyze a Retention Problem

1. Ask these key questions:
   Is there really a problem? When did it start? Are only certain shifts or job categories affected? How bad is it? Is it getting better or worse? Are there manifestations that suggest a general morale problem? What is the underlying cause or causes? What has been our response to date?
2. Determine the turnover rate for your organization, your department, each shift, and each job classification. Normally, rates are higher for night shifts and nonexempt workers such as phlebotomists and clerks. Use this formula to calculate turnover rate:

$$\frac{\text{total number of resignations per year}}{\text{average number of employees}} \times 100.$$

3. Consider these possible causes:
   Lack of competitive pay, poor benefits, poor work environment, poor location, inadequate parking, or other external factors.
   Weak recruiting and selection process.
   Inadequate orientation and training program.
   Lack of supervisory support.
4. Gather information from these sources:
   Newly hired persons or candidates. Ask what attracted them, and what they like or dislike about the job and the workplace.
   Employees who request transfers.
   Recruiters or recruitment-retention committees.
   Exit interviews.
5. List the financial incentives offered by your organization and its competitors.

1. Overqualified or underqualified
2. Difficulty in getting along with superiors
3. Strong aversion to overtime, changes, or irregular schedules
4. Greater interest in rewards than in responsibilities
5. Tendency to be inflexible, intolerant, or strongly opinionated
6. Supersensitive; unable to handle criticism
7. Strong likes and dislikes
8. Left previous jobs for "personal reasons"
9. Inability to cope with stress or difficult people
10. Changed schools and jobs frequently

Figure 16.1   Ten strong signs of susceptibility to turnover.

6. Reflect on how you promote the jobs to candidates during employment interviews.
7. Study your indoctrination process and determine how it affects new trainees.
8. Consider your coaching ability and team-building skill.

Recruiting and selecting personnel

When your interviewing and selection process works correctly, people will stay for a long time.[6]

A good recruiting and selecting strategy seeks employees who are customer-oriented. By attracting employees who share the philosophy and goals of an organization, and by achieving better employee-job fits, retention is improved. Internal sources are the best because the candidates already are familiar with the organizational culture, so any disillusionment after the hiring is less likely.[6]

Potential quitters can often be spotted by reviewing employment histories and asking a few provocative questions. We seldom hire "new" employees. Most are "used" employees—they have had previous jobs. If they have not stayed long at previous places of employment, the likelihood that they will be with you for a long time is not great.

During the interview look for the signs of turnover susceptibility listed in Figure 16.1. Questions that help detect potential quitters are shown in Figure 16.2.

Special Notes

Stop, look, and listen when discussing the reasons why a candidate has elected to change employers. Watch facial expressions and body language.

1. How would you . . . (invite responses to relevant professional or technical questions).
2. Tell me how you would . . . (describe a relevant interpersonal conflict or sensitive issue).
3. What kind of people do you find difficult to work with? Why?
4. What assignments, policies, or kinds of supervision annoy you?
5. What do you want to be doing 5 years from now?
6. What concerns you the most about being able to handle this job?
7. What kind of loyalty does an organization owe its employees?
8. What kind of loyalty does an employee owe his or her employer?
9. If you could change the job being offered, what would you change?
10. What are your strongest assets?

Figure 16.2 Interview questions that may detect potential dropouts.

Be suspicious of lateral moves or signs of immaturity such as chronic dissatisfaction, inability to cope with stressful situations, or rationalizing failures.

Be wary of those who leave "for personal reasons" or who are reluctant to discuss previous resignations.

INDOCTRINATION OF NEW EMPLOYEES

The Texas Instrument Company reduced its turnover by 40%, and Corning Glass Works slashed theirs by 69% simply by improving their orientation program. [7] The highest turnover rates are during the first year of employment. The three factors affected by the indoctrination process are (1) the ability of the employee to handle the work, (2) a sense of belonging, and (3) supervisory support.

THE COACHING PROCESS

Coaching is face-to-face leadership. It means paying attention to people. Good coaches are enthusiastic leaders who push people to the limits of their capability, but not to a level of discouragement.

Winning coaches know that today's employees want more than a job. They want meaningful work. They want to know not only what, when, where and who, but also WHY. They want some say in HOW they do their work. They do not want to be managed, they want to be led.

Situational leadership is the key to good coaching. The coach knows the motivational needs of each subordinate, and responds appropriately.

Different strokes for different folks.

"Go-getters" want challenge and promotions. "Old faithfuls" want security, friendship, and a pleasant work environment. The "turn-me-loose" ones crave free expression and the opportunity for innovation and creativity.

A winning coach's attitude is "How can I help," not "You're doing that wrong."

Great coaches practice managing by walking around (MBWA). Like athletic coaches, they do not manage from offices; they are out where the action is. MBWA is being where you are needed, when you are needed. It is not looking for something to complain about. It is not rambling around saying "How'ya doin."

Practitioners of MBWA are facilitators, source persons, helpers, defenders, and cheerleaders. They are perceived by subordinates as bosses help them get their job done, not get in their way, harp, or nitpick.

Nitpickers end up having to pick new employees.

Winning coaches delegate, not dump. They know the difference between delegating and making busywork. They get people to solve their own problems, thereby making them more self-sufficient. They permit their associates to make on-the-spot decisions that affect customers.

As cheerleaders, coaches know when and how to praise. They praise work that is outstanding, work that is improving, and work that is always finished on time. They cheer loudly and publicly when a teammate comes up with an innovative suggestion.

These managers do not praise when the praise is not sincere, when it is manipulative, when it is not earned, when it would be excessive, or when it would embarrass.

Coaches also know how to, and how not to, find fault. They eschew global criticism, being very specific about what they fault. They address behavior or results, not personality or attitude.

Coaches support and defend their staffs. Baseball managers know the importance of this. They rush out onto the field to protest an umpire's call, even when they know the call is correct. Laboratory coaches intercede when their associates are attacked by angry customers.

How to Decrease Turnover Through Team Building

Turnover is lower in closely knit groups.[8] Since loyalty locks people into place, it follows that team building can be a powerful force in any retention strategy.

Two major motivational needs that are satisfied by team membership are the need for affiliation and the need for achievement. Students or employees with limited skills may derive their satisfaction from team achievements. For individuals who earn formal or informal leadership roles on the team, the motivational desire for power or control is satiated.

A strong indoctrination program gets the team-building process off to a good start. Experts match each team member's strengths and interests with his or her assigned tasks, thus taking advantage of strengths, and making weaknesses irrelevant.

How to Avert Resignations

Susceptibility to turnover is much higher in certain job or employee categories. A person who will soon be eligible for retirement is very turnover-resistant. On the other hand, experienced technologists may be very restless unless their jobs provide satisfactory rewards and interest. The key to preventing resignations is to recognize the signs of restlessness, not wait for the fait accompli. This calls for an active strategy.

The "Proactive" Strategy

There is a big difference between "proactive" leaders and those reactive leaders who practice crisis management. Proactive leaders anticipate problems by detecting and correcting areas of concern before these concerns develop into problems. They know their staffers well and have close daily contact. They know the susceptible ones and have sensitive antennae for dissatisfaction.

Telltale signs of possible resignations include escalation of complaints, decline in the willingness to volunteer for special assignments, and loss of interest in daily routines. Potential exiters miss or avoid meetings. When they do show up, they maintain a stony silence, or voice only negative comments. Their silence at meetings contrasts with their constant harping in the corridors. They spend little time discussing professional activities or technical problems. They are not interested in new departmental plans, equipment, or methods. Resistance to change stiffens.

Avoidance tactics such as taking more and longer breaks, arriving late, and leaving early are used frequently. Sick leave may be abused, absences from work stations may occur often.

The potential quitters constantly relate how much better things are elsewhere. If their coworkers maintain a positive attitude toward work and employer, the discontented ones either fall silent or try to proselytize the others. They interrupt their conversations with coworkers and look embarrassed when their boss approaches.

Finally, when employees start showing up for work unusually well dressed and say they have dental appointments, or when they take long lunch breaks, they may be interviewing for other jobs. This is even more likely if they make many telephone calls from outside the laboratory.

Quitters Still may be Undecided

Often employees have mixed feelings about leaving, and are struggling to arrive at a definite decision. They are trying to convince themselves that things are better elsewhere. To do that, they exaggerate the positives of new jobs and the negatives of their current ones. *Your approach is to play on these doubts.*

Too often, supervisors write employees off at this point. A cool or critical attitude on the part of the supervisor reinforces the employees' dissatisfaction and encourages them to leave. So does eliminating them from participation in group activities. Faced with employees who now have negative attitudes, there is a natural tendency for supervisors to move into an avoidance pattern. One laboratory manager, when informed that a member of her supervisory staff was job hunting, called him in, pointed her finger at him, and accused him of disloyalty. Then she told him that he was "excused" from her weekly staff meetings. Guess how long it took him to resign!

Psychiatrists warn that when depressed people stop talking about suicide it often means that they have made the decision to take their lives. Likewise, when an employee suddenly stops complaining, he may have changed his mind, but more likely has made a commitment to leave.

What to do When a Resignation Appears Imminent

When an employee's behavior reveals the telltale signs of quitting, critique your coaching of her by asking yourself these questions:

What are her motivational needs?
What have I done to help her meet these needs?
Have I made her job more challenging, but still doable?
When I delegate to her, do I give her enough authority to do the job?
What have I done to increase, or at least preserve, her self-esteem?
Has my praise-criticism ratio been high?
What specific things did I do that could have impaired our relationship?

After you have analyzed the situation, draw up a remedial plan and start fence mending.

A Letter of Resignation is on Your Desk. Now What?

Stop what you are doing. Sit down and ask the employee why she is quitting. Let her talk. Do not interrupt. After she has gone through all her reasons (they may not be good ones), ask a lot of questions, including the critical one: what is the real reason she is pulling up stakes? The truth will emerge if your rapport is reasonably good.

Remember that our approach is to play on doubts. Ask questions about the new job. What new responsibilities will the employee have? How much of a salary increase? What aspects of the job concern her? What obstacles are anticipated? How does her family feel about the move? You may be the only person to whom she will reveal her concerns about her ability to handle the new job.

Look for the possibilities in the old job. Discuss the person's future with your organization in frank terms. One of the most important leadership skills is persuasiveness. Here is the ultimate challenge to use it. You may be able to negotiate relatively minor concessions to persuade her to stay. Offer a transfer or reassignment.

Ask her to hold off a final decision. Check with your boss to see what could be worked out to keep her. When all else fails, leave the door open for her to return.

Let her know that she would be welcomed back ("I'll hold your position open for 1 month. This will give you time to determine if you like the new job.").

Do Not Forget the Stayers

The other employees will watch these events with great interest. When one person finds a new job, it reminds other employees that they too have choices. They tend to grow restless. However, if a person moves into an entirely new vocation, the change is less contagious than when the move is merely to a different employer.

Those who stay also note how you treat the "lame duck." If that treatment is unfavorable, those who leave at a later date will keep it secret up to the last moment.

REFERENCES

1. Davidow WH, Uttal B: *Total Customer Service*. New York, Harper & Row, 1989.
2. Mercer MW: Turnover: Reducing the Costs. *Personnel* 1988;65:36–42.
3. Prescott PA, Bower SA: Controlling nursing turnover. *Nurs Manage* 1987;18:60.
4. Zaradona JL, Camuso MA: A study of exit interviews: Does the last word count? *Personnel* 1985;62:47–48.
5. Kerfoot K: Retention: What's it all about? *Nurs Econ* 1988;6:42–43.
6. Goldzimer LS: *'I'm First': Your Customer's Message to You*. New York, Rawson Associates, 1989.
7. Zemke R: Employee orientation: A process, not a program. *Training* 1989;26:33–40.
8. Strauss G, Sayles LR: *Personnel: the Human Problems of Management*, ed 3. Englewood Cliffs, NJ, Prentice-Hall, 1972.

17. Improving Productivity

MANAGING A LABORATORY can be compared with managing a restaurant in which all the customers are seated as trios. The first customer orders the food (the physician), the second customer eats the food (the patient), and the third customer picks up the tab (whoever pays the hospital bill). In this chapter we focus on satisfying that third customer.

WHAT IS PRODUCTIVITY?

On a statistical basis, productivity is defined as the number of output units divided by the number of input units.

In general it is better to raise productivity by increasing the output rather than decreasing the input. Lowering input by cutting back work hours or using cheaper reagents affects the service quality, and quality must be factored in. Doing things right the first time avoids the time-consuming tasks of correcting mistakes and reassuring unhappy clients.

Laboratory managers must maintain a balance between productivity and quality. If turnaround time always has priority over attention to patients' comfort, then customer satisfaction is ill served. For example, a phlebotomist is confronted by a confused, weeping patient. Should that phlebotomist pause to console the patient or hurry to get the blood specimens back to the laboratory on time?

When managers are clear, specific, and consistent about relative priorities, then conflict between productivity and customer service will disappear.[1] Productivity involves both efficiency and effectiveness. Efficiency is doing things right, and effectiveness is doing the right things.

THE TWO STRATEGIC OBJECTIVES

In sociotechnical systems such as laboratories, every job is a combination of two considerations. One is the best technical system for being productive, the other is the best social organization for bringing human resources to bear on that technology.[2]

The two objectives for reaching our goal of higher productivity are (1) to make it possible for employees to accomplish more and (2) to make employees want to accomplish more.

EXTRINSIC BARRIERS TO PRODUCTIVITY

The extrinsic factors reside in an organization's infrastructure—the necessary human and physical resources such as skills, materials, technologies, strategies, procedures, finance, logistics, and technology.[3] There is no point in addressing issues of motivation, participation, and creativity if the people and tools are inadequate for the job.[3] The strategy related to the infrastructure is clear—remove all the barriers to productivity.

Comments on Productivity

Following are some comments that you might hear from a group of clinical laboratory inspectors returning from a survey. They illustrate some of the many extrinsic barriers to productivity.

Physical Layout

"The guys who designed that lab never heard of work flow."

Equipment

"Their new multitest chemical analyzer is fantastic, and they have a backup instrument for every test."

Supplies

"Can you believe that they're still making their own bacteriologic media?"

Communication System

"I wish we had their LIS system."

Interdepartmental Rapport

"Rapport with the nursing service is bad. They waste a lot of time smoothing ruffled feathers. I overheard a lot of bickering and angry comments." "Yeah, and they spend lots of time investigating incident reports and complaints. But at least they do record them."

Environmental Control

"No wonder they have a high turnover. The place is hot, noisy, and uninviting."

Parking

"I noticed that there is reserved parking for patients and blood donors."

Staffing and Schedules

"They rotate their day and evening people, use part-timers to balance work loads, and they really go all out for crosstraining. Techs, not supervisors, prepare vacation and holiday schedules."

Policies

"Those poor techs are hamstrung by some pretty stupid rules and policies. For instance, they still require a doctor's certification for every 1-day absence."

Interruptions

"Do you know how many times my discussion with the chemistry supervisor was interrupted?"

Work Load

"With all those empty beds and fixed costs, how do they survive?"

In a 1989 survey, 428 laboratorians reported on factors that lowered productivity. The three factors mentioned most frequently (over 50% of respondents) were inefficient test-ordering patterns, stat abuse, and understaffing. At the lower end of this list (less than 10%) were unions, poor inventory control or inadequate performance standards.[4]

INTRINSIC BARRIERS TO PRODUCTIVITY

Intrinsic barriers result from motivation, and are therefore less susceptible to objective evaluation. It is relatively simple to spot and to do something about malfunctioning equipment, but how about getting Alice to show up on time, Louise to take fewer sick days, Bob to make fewer errors, and Steve to spend less time talking about sports?

Every group establishes its own productivity norms by applying the principles of convergence and conformity.[2] Once a norm is established, it is difficult to elevate it. Any member who departs from the group's norm, whether up or down, will be pressured by the other group members to conform.[2]

Relying on power and authority to change norms can be risky. Over and above the resistance that will be provoked, there is the likelihood of alienating those who are expected to alter their behavior. These people become resentful and even vengeful.[2]

Overreliance on output standards may not be conducive to higher productivity because those responsible for attaining the standards often have little "ownership" of the goal since they had no say in developing it.[5] In Chapter 14 ("Introducing Change") we mentioned the importance of employee input in the formulation of standards.

According to Fitz-Enz,[6] white-collar productivity correlates closely with self-esteem, responsibility, coworker relationships, and competency, as well as the availability of resources. The so-called quality of work life approach[2] attempts to better productivity through worker participation.

HOW TO INVESTIGATE A PRODUCTIVITY PROBLEM

Productivity Comparisons

Only 50% of clinical laboratories measure productivity.[4] Most laboratories that do so rely on the CAP Workload Reporting System or some equivalent. Once managers understand the shortcomings and pitfalls of these systems, they usually find them useful, especially for comparing their productivity with that of similar laboratories.

Output can be measured in terms of billable units. For example, if we replace a procedure that requires duplicate test runs with one that does not, standard work units increase, but billable units stay the same. Thus, billable units are more representative of productivity. On the other hand, non–revenue-producing activities such as teaching, record keeping, and research and development take their toll of productivity when these statistics are based exclusively on billable test units.

Staffing Ratios

In 1989, the average hospital laboratory had one technical full-time equivalent for every seven occupied beds.[4] When adjusted to reflect outpatient visits, an acceptable ratio is one full-time equivalent to 3.5 to 4.5 adjusted occupied beds, according to Barros.[7]

Work Flow Patterns

Study of detailed work flow charts may reveal steps that could be eliminated or modified, or work stations that could be rearranged. These charts should highlight steps during which the operator is not operating (eg, during centrifugation or incubation), or is waiting for other workers to complete preliminary activities. In some laboratories there is more socializing around centrifuges and copy machines than around water fountains.

While waiting for blood collectors to return, some waiting technicians grab collection trays and go out to help the collectors. Some busy themselves with work details, and some just stand around and gab. What they do is what they have been taught to do and what is tolerated.

Time Studies

Each employee maintains a daily time log in which are recorded activities at 15- to 30-minute intervals for at least 1 week, and preferably longer. These records often reveal an embarrassing amount of time wasted, even by the people who complain so bitterly about being overworked. On the other hand, the charts may substantiate complaints about missed breaks or meetings, or harassment by visitors such as sales representatives. Even if productivity does not increase as the result of such studies, the effort is always worthwhile because it teaches the employees a lot about their time-management skills.

Productivity of supervisors, managers, and staff professionals should also be measured. Too often, only the front-line workers are considered.[5]

Input from Employees

When efficiency or an efficiency expert is mentioned, employees get upset. They fear job elimination or think that they are being accused of being inefficient. Before soliciting an efficiency expert's input, it is advisable to make it clear to your employees that you want to help them spend less time on the boring or trying aspects of their work so they have more time to work on the things they like to do or that will enhance their careers.

Staff surveys can pinpoint trouble spots. Roseman[8] describes a simple, practical questionnaire for this purpose. It focuses primarily on supervisory support and expectations, communication, freedom to act, and training opportunities.

TAKING ACTION

The more thorough the study of the problem, the more corrective options that will become apparent. Barros[9] recommends a three-pronged approach. The first consists of getting a handle on the statistical analyses. The second is correcting infrastructure problems such as instrumentation, reagents, physical layout, position descriptions, policies, and indoctrination. The third addresses supervisory weaknesses.

Decrease Input Time

Laboratory input is the selection and ordering of tests by the clinical staff. The following actions or devices address this activity:

Update manuals for requesting services.
Redesign request forms.
Computerize.
Use pneumatic tubes for specimen and report delivery.
Increase speed and frequency of blood collections.

Decrease Output Time

Output is the transmission of reports from the laboratory to the clinicians who ordered the tests. The following items are related to output: design of report forms, computers and pneumatic tubes, telephone reports (especially stats and panic values), and attachment of reports to charts.

Test More Efficiently

More efficient testing may be accomplished by using better instrumentation and automation, asking for fewer stats and repeated tests, and requesting fewer quality control tests when quality is not noticeably lower.

Sometimes we can learn from our "lazy" techs. Most of their shortcuts are acceptable as well as practical. Adopt what is good, and make them stop doing what is bad.

Reduce Staff

Productivity is increased by "down sizing" only when the work load is not also reduced. As mentioned before, it is usually better to increase the work load rather than decrease the number of workers. However, both actions may be feasible.

Reduce the number of managers and poorly utilized specialists by increasing the span of control of those remaining, delegating administrative chores to techs, and discontinuing marginal services.

Automate.

Refer out tests that cannot be processed efficiently because of low volume, lack of time, or special expertise.

Get rid of poor performers. The manager who tolerates an unsatisfactory performer who cannot or will not change is unfair to that individual and to the organization.

Motivate

A commonly stated tenet is that working harder will not significantly increase productivity in the long haul. That may be true of work units that are already functioning at or near capacity. Study after study, however, has disclosed that most employees work far below their potential. If we can motivate these people, a significant long-term increase in productivity can be achieved. We have all witnessed the remarkable improvement that takes place when an incompetent leader is replaced by a competent one.

According to Misschkind,[3] the three pillars of motivation are desire, self-confidence, and commitment. The three factors form an interactive system, each affecting the others.

Here are the motivational factors most commonly mentioned in the literature[6,7,10] as affecting productivity favorably:

Assigning productivity a high priority
Feedback and recognition
Job performance feedback
Job opportunities
Networking
Planning as a team
Education and training
Communication (keeping everyone informed)
Involving employees in decision making
Raising performance standards
Strengthening training programs
Upgrading performance rewards
Improving general supervision
Rewarding and celebrating success

Mention already has been made of the importance of group norms, and the difficulty of altering these. Norms can be altered successfully through the following actions:

1. Point out that the purpose of the change is to make your employees' jobs easier and more fulfilling, not to eliminate positions.
2. Get your employees involved and enthusiastic. The use of quality circles is an effective way to achieve this.
3. If an efficiency expert or time-study specialist is brought in, promise your employees that the expert has no power, but is only there to advise.
4. State that the employees will make the changes.
5. Describe as specifically as possible the direct and indirect benefits of the changes.

Encourage Innovation

The challenge to management is to maintain productivity through creative approaches to work assignments that maximize human and machine resources.[11] Reward ideas for improving work procedures or enhancing revenues.[7] Reinforce model traits such as willingness to change traditional behavior and take risks.[7]

Results of Programs to Increase Productivity

Cole[12] reported that his efforts achieved not only increased productivity, but also fewer clerical errors, less delays, fewer stat orders and telephone calls, and shorter inpatient stays.

Hallam's[4] survey found that the productivity-enhancing measures that worked best were improved instrumentation, automation, computerization, and schedule changes. The least successful were salary increases or incentives, staffing cuts, and curbing stat abuse.

REFERENCES

1. Goldzimer LS: *'I'm First': Your Customer's Message to You*. New York, Rawson Associates, 1989.

2. Blake R, Mouton JS: *Productivity: The Human Side*. New York, AMACOM Book Division, 1981.

3. Misschkind LA: Seven steps to productivity improvement. *Personnel* 1987; 64:22–30.

4. Hallam K: Laboratory productivity. *MLO* 1989;21:22–31.

5. Midas MT Jr, Werther W Jr: Productivity: The missing link in corporate strategy. *Manage Rev* 74:3 March 1985;74:44–48.

6. Fitz-Enz J: White-collar productivity: The employees' side. *Manage Rev* 1986;75:52.

7. Barros A: Improving productivity: The administrator's point of view. *MLO* 1990;22:21–22.

8. Roseman E: How to improve your lab's productivity. *MLO* 1984;16:51–54.

9. Barros A: Identifying the causes of low productivity. *MLO* 1988;20:37–40.

10. Deeprose D: Three key elements of a productivity improvement program. *Supervis Manage* 1989;34:7–11.

11. Schein E: Organizational culture. *Am Psychologist* 1990;45:109.

12. Cole BW: Improving lab utilization through test profiles. *MLO* 1982;14:21–38.

18. Budgeting and Cost Containment

THIS CHAPTER IS also dedicated to those laboratorians who must satisfy the clients who pay the bills. We will not describe how to perform the necessary cost-accounting procedures (see the referenced books and articles for that). We will touch on those activities with which laboratory supervisors and managers should be familiar, and we will suggest some practical cost-containment measures.

Supervisors and managers must have a practical grasp of cost accounting and budget preparation; technical and professional expertise is insufficient in today's laboratories.[1] Where do laboratory employees acquire these skills? Many enroll in formal educational programs; others attend selected seminars and workshops. A few, like Lucia Berte,[2] take the initiative and organize an in-house program for all supervisory personnel.

Because of the 1982 Tax Equity and Fiscal Responsibility Act and the switch to prospective Medicare payment, the laboratory is becoming a major cost center and a smaller generator of revenue. Under prospective payment, tests for Medicare inpatients simply add to laboratory and hospital expenses.

MAJOR ACCOUNTING DOCUMENTS

Balance Sheet

The balance sheet is a summary of the institution's financial position as of the date listed. It lists the assets and the liabilities, and these must balance, hence the name of the document.

Income Statement

The income statement shows what revenues have been added and what expenses have been subtracted. The result is net income.

Budget

Clear, detailed, financial records are necessary for several purposes, the primary one being budget preparation and acceptance. Not all records are easy to maintain. For example, the finance department uses different time segments for various cost-accounting activities. Payroll data are usually tallied in 2- or 4-week periods, while most other statistics are accumulated monthly. As a result, it is often necessary to manipulate the figures to derive the information needed.[3]

Budgets serve first as a financial plan for some future period; second, they are a tool for controlling costs during the period covered by that budget plan. The better their planning and preparation, the easier it is to get them accepted, and to stay within their limits.

Used as a control mechanism, a budget is a cost-containment aid that helps keep expenditures in line with available resources. Through monthly review of the plan, deviations can be identified by comparing the budgeted and actual costs. Significant variances must be analyzed so that corrective action can be undertaken. It is this cost-containment aspect that is so important to administrators, third-party payers, and the patients who are concerned about the costs of medical care.

Budget changes may be needed for a number of reasons, eg, improved products become available, work load changes, or equipment fails or becomes too costly to repair, all before anticipated dates.[4]

Forecasting

One of the tools used for budgets is "forecasting," which is looking ahead to predict what will be happening 2, 5, or 10 years down the road. Trends are noted in the testing service, patient population, and medical staff. Annual salary increases, increases in supply expenses, and possible changes in work loads are also considered.

Kinds of Budgets

There are three kinds of budgets: the (fixed or flexible) operating budget, with its statistical, expense, and revenue components; the capital budget; and the cash budget.

Laboratory participation in statistical, revenue, and cash budgets is usually limited to providing operational statistics. Much more laboratory effort goes into departmental expense and capital expenditure budgets. These must be clearly documented to withstand scrutiny by institutional administrators, and government and accrediting agency representatives. Federal and state governments impose many standards and regulations on hospital budgets. Third-party payers impose additional requirements, as does the JCAHO.[4]

Responsibility Budgeting

Responsibility budgeting is a system that relates the responsibility for expenses to the people who cause them to be incurred. There are five basic concepts.[5]

1. Expenses are charged to the lowest-level unit that can incur them.
2. Only items that can be controlled by that unit are included.
3. The unit must be headed by someone who is held responsible for expenditures by that unit.
4. Every item can be controlled by someone in the unit.
5. The unit chief agrees that the planned expenditure is realistic.

Budgetary Inputs

Typical internal budgetary input[6]:

test cost
work load statistics
income or revenue (past, present, and projected)
cost of capital equipment (initial cost, life expectancy, and yearly depreciation)
operating expenses for reagents, expendables, service contracts, and other items
personnel (present and projected)

Typical external budgetary input:

average daily patient census with breakdowns by case mix and acuity levels
projected service expansion or service reduction plans
contractual payment levels (Medicare, Medicaid, and self-pay)
projections of changes in reimbursement schedules

Laboratory budget summary[3]:

Narrative description of budget
Condensed income statement for the budget period
Summary of capital expenditure requests
Cash flow analysis
Key factors used in forecasting
Estimates of the impact of the budget on the institution's services and finances

EXPENSES

The key aspect of analyzing financial statements is the evaluation of costs. Here is one classification of expenditures:

Basic Expenses

salaries
supplies

Allocated Expenses

phlebotomy costs
reference laboratory
office
equipment maintenance
depreciation
education
other

Indirect Expenses

institutional
laboratory

Capital Expenditures

Load the justification guns with dollar signs and the quality of patient care — the ammunition that makes the loudest bang.[4]

The acquisition of equipment demands that cost be balanced against need. It is not enough to prove that the equipment will lighten the work load or increase accuracy. While these factors do enter into the final decision to acquire or not to acquire, the primary consideration is whether there is actually a need for additional equipment.[4]

You must know when a piece of equipment represents a capital expenditure. This is based on its cost and its expected useful life.[4] Each organization establishes its own figures for what is called a capital expenditure.[4]

Obsolescence should not be based only on the age of the instrument. Downtime, quality control costs, and reliability must also be considered.

Most capital budget requests are subject to several levels of review and approval. Ensure that the following information is provided on any request[3]:

replacement or new item
justification and realistic assessment of urgency or priority
detailed projection of all costs
impact on revenues, if any

Dozens of questions must be answered in any justification for a capital expenditure. Here are just a few:

What is the start-up time?
What are the stat capabilities?

How much space is needed?

Will changes in plumbing or electrical service be required?

Can it be interfaced with the computer?

What sample size is necessary?

What is the cost of the instrument, supplies, and labor?

What is its service record?

Most organizations have special procedures and forms for this purpose. If you want to receive your share of the hospital's budget, be familiar with this procedure, including the deadlines for filing.

Operating Ratio Formulas

Ratios provide quantitative information about supply and labor usage, productivity, efficiency, and break-even volumes—data that help control costs and improve service.[7] Figure 18.1 shows some of the more frequently used ratios.

Calculation of Cost of New Procedures

The data needed for determination of cost per test include time and hourly rate of labor (tech, aide, clerical), cost of controls and standards, and the indirect expenses.[8]

These costs are usually calculated only for high-volume tests and instruments. In many laboratories, a few automated instruments and manual procedures account for most of the work load. Thus, detailed costs need only be calculated for these.[8]

Determining Charges for Tests

There is no longer much direct relationship between billable and payable tests, another consequence of the shift to prospective pricing. However, laboratories still list their charges for those who do still pay what is asked.

Once the cost per test has been determined, the charge is easily pegged at a percentage markup, eg, 10%. However, charges are often based not on the cost of performing the tests, but on what the competition charges, or the ceilings imposed by payers or regulatory agencies.

COST CONTAINMENT

A tight budget brings out the best creative instincts.[9]

Supervisors are key instigators of cost reductions because they can suggest means of cost reduction as well as oversee the implementation and measurement of these ideas. They also have a direct influence over many costs. When supervisors are cost conscious, it is reflected in the behavior of their employees.

Costs can be reduced in three major ways: (1) by producing the same or increased output with a smaller staff budget, (2) by reducing other costs, and (3) by decreasing the number of tests per patient.[10]

$$\text{CAP units/worked hours} = \frac{\text{CAP work units}}{\text{worked hours}}$$

$$\text{Percent productivity} = \frac{\text{work units/worked hours}}{60}$$

$$\text{Needed work hours} = \frac{\text{work units/month}}{45 \times 173.33*}$$

$$\text{FTEs needed} = \frac{\text{needed work hours}}{80\dagger}$$

$$\text{Supply cost/test} = \frac{\text{supply costs}}{\text{billable procedures}}$$

$$\text{Labor cost/test} = \frac{\text{labor cost}}{\text{billable procedures}}$$

$$\text{Productivity/FTE hour} = \frac{\text{billable procedures}}{\text{FTEs} \times 40 \times 52}$$

$$\text{Direct cost/test} = \frac{\text{direct costs}}{\text{billable procedures}}$$

$$\text{Total cost/test} = \frac{\text{total costs}}{\text{billable procedures}}$$

$$\text{Efficiency ratio} = \frac{\text{productivity/FTE hour} \times 100}{\text{direct cost/test}}$$

$$\text{Variable cost/test} = \frac{\text{supplies} + \frac{1}{2}\text{ labor cost}}{\text{billable procedures}}$$

$$\text{Fixed cost/test} = \frac{\text{allocated expenses} + \frac{1}{2}\text{ labor cost}}{\text{billable procedues}}$$

$$\text{Revenue/test} = \frac{\text{revenue}}{\text{billable procedures}}$$

$$\text{Break-even volume} = \frac{\text{fixed costs}}{(\text{revenue/test} - \text{variable cost per test})}$$

Figure 18.1 Ratios useful in the budgeting process.[7,10] FTE indicates full-time equivalent. *National average work units/hours. 173.33 is the number of hours worked in a standard month. †Number of hours authorized per pay period for FTE based on 2-week pay period, or 26 pay periods per year.

Use of Ratios to Focus on Problems

Fantus[11] found paydirt by using a few ratios of fiscal statistics to compare his laboratory's performance with that of other laboratories. In Figure 18.2, the "standards" represent the average percentages in the laboratories surveyed by Fantus.

Reducing Staff Budget

Townsend[9] writes that man simplifies only when under pressure. "Put him under financial pressure. He will scream in anguish, then come up with a plan which is

Ratio	Standard
Labor	
labor costs/net sales	Less than 40%
Supplies	
supply costs/net sales	Less than 15%
Indirect costs	
indirect costs/net sales	Less than 35%

Figure 18.2   Example of how to use ratios to evaluate productivity.[10]

not only less expensive, but is also faster and better than his original proposal, which you sent back."

1. Increase automation and computerization.
2. Replace technologists with technicians and aides. The jury is still out on this practice. It has led to mixed results in the past, with extreme variations among hospitals.[10] However, the use of less qualified people to perform simple tasks makes sense and relieves technologists of boring tasks.
3. Reduce salaries or benefits. Many institutions have been cutting back on benefits, especially health benefits. However, niggardly reward practices are usually counterproductive.[10]
4. Improve productivity. Effective leadership can reduce labor costs. Take a close look at where salaried funds go (Figure 18.3). Each of the activities directly associated with work bears scrutiny, as do idle times during analytical processes. Simple observation readily detects abuse of breaks or time wasted during centrifugation or incubation.
5. Schedule for efficiency. Redistribute personnel or work among shifts. Look at vacations and other schedules. Organize daily work loads more efficiently. Make better use of part-time employees and volunteers. Look into flexible scheduling.
6. Cross train. Have backups for each work station. Do not be hamstrung by absences or workload variances.

Reducing Other Costs

Besides labor, the principal costs are materials and instruments. Costs in the following five categories can be reduced.

1. Supplies and Reagents

There are opportunities for savings through tougher purchasing practices. Savings can also be attained by guarding against outdating and other forms of reagent and supply waste.[10]

```
        I. Paid time off
       II. Worked hours
           A. Workloaded activities
              1. Analytical time
              2. Idle time
           B. Non-workloaded activities
              1. Administrative
              2. Clerical
              3. Educational
              4. Break time
```

Figure 18.3 Personnel paid hours.

2. Equipment and Instruments

Should you buy, lease, or rent? Prospective payment is changing the relative advantages and disadvantages of instrument acquisition alternatives.[10] Comparison shopping for the best deal is worth the time and effort.

3. Reference Laboratory Fees

We have two options here. The first is to find a less expensive reference laboratory. The second, and more difficult, is to discourage test-order abuses by clinicians. This is, of course, one important aspect of utilization review.

4. Quality-Control Costs

Sharp[7] claims that almost one fourth of analytical costs are attributable to "quality costs," which he defines as those of controls, standards, repeats, calibrations, and correcting report errors. Improved assays or instrumentation can reduce some of these costs. He cites an example of time and cost saved by eliminating the need for running duplicate radioimmunoassay determinations after introducing a self-calibrating instrument.[7]

5. Other Costs

Fiscally alert managers can find other ways to lower expenditures. For example, Nelson[12] reported on the use of a cash award suggestion system that yielded ideas that saved over $100,000 within 1 month.[12]

Take a close look at your educational costs, but hesitate before making cuts in this essential activity. In fact, during times of change, educational activities warrant increased attention and administrative support. However, most programs can be streamlined, with resulting savings and no loss of quality.

Educational endeavors include orientation programs. The higher your department's turnover, the more costly indoctrination programs become. These periods of intensive training must be designed expertly and conducted competently if they are to be cost-effective.

Specialists and Researchers

In some laboratories, research, paper writing, and educational activities may take big bites out of the laboratory budget. Many of these activities may be of no or marginal benefit to the laboratory or the institution. Laboratory scientists may have more loyalty to their specialty group than to their employer or their clients. It may be necessary to reevaluate the priorities of the people so engaged.

Reduce the Number of Tests per Inpatient

1. Decrease unnecessary tests and transfusions. Laboratory services to inpatients can be reduced; the challenge is to cut only the services that have little or no effect on patient outcome.

   In concert with other physicians, laboratory medical directors initiate and maintain dialogues regarding laboratory cost v clinical benefit trade-offs. Together they reeducate clinicians about relevant tests and how to eliminate less effective procedures from their practices.[10] Similar savings can be realized through more judicious control of the use of blood products.

   Gore[13] reported that showing physicians their patients' laboratory bills and corresponding payments from Medicare resulted in fewer tests being ordered.

   One must guard against going overboard on test restrictions. Blind refusal to add useful tests to the menu, restricted hours of operation, and slow response to stat orders may lengthen patient stays and increase the cost of some cases.[10]

2. Improve use of admission testing. More intensive discriminate use of admission profiles, diagnosis-related group ordering profiles, and interpretive algorithms can cut costs by reducing the length of the hospital stay, often with better patient outcome. On the other hand, profiles of *indiscriminate* design and use are another matter. They are ripe for curtailment with minimal negative impact on patient outcome.[10]

3. Decrease stat order and other special order turnaround times. Indiscriminate stat ordering should be suspected when such requests constitute more than 15% of day work and more than 35% of evening work. This may not be the fault of the ordering clinicians. It may result from poor routine laboratory service.

   Abuses of other requests for special handling, such as demands that reports be ready by a designated time, should be corrected. Preventable late presurgical admissions and overuse by fledgling housestaff members are not uncommon and can be both costly and frustrating to laboratory personnel.

An *MLO* survey[14] found that the most successful cost-control measures were: creative buying (17%), group purchasing (16%), scheduling staff or work load (11%), and inventory control (10%).

Improved laboratory utilization and new technology were offered as the most promising cost-control avenues, while ill-advised cost cuts included staff cuts, needed capital purchases not made, and continuing education cutbacks.[14]

REFERENCES

1. Barros A: Financial management is more than monitoring a budget. *MLO* 1988;20:43–47.

2. Berte LM: Financial skills for the non-financial manager. *MLO* 1989;21:39–42.

3. McConnell CR: *The Effective Health Care Supervisor*, ed 2. Rockville, MD, Aspen Publishers Inc, 1988.

4. Sattler J: *A Practical Guide to Financial Management of the Clinical Laboratory*. Oradell, NJ, Medical Economics Books, 1980.

5. Bennington JL: *Management and Cost Control Techniques for the Clinical Laboratory*. Baltimore, University Park Press, 1977.

6. Bender JL: Guidelines for laboratory administration: III. *MLO* 1984;16:83–87.

7. Sharp JW: A cost-accounting system targeted to DRGs. *MLO* 1985;17:34–41.

8. Haughney JD: Test cost analysis: More vital than ever. In Fitzgibbon R, Statland BE (eds): *DRG Survival Manual for the Clinical Lab*. Oradell, NJ, Medical Economics Books, 1985, chap 4.

9. Townsend R: *Up the Organization*. New York, Fawcett World Library, 1970.

10. Johnson JL: A cost-cutting strategy. In Fitzgibbon R, Statland BE (eds): *DRG Survival Manual for the Clinical Lab*. Oradell, NJ, Medical Economics Books, 1985:74.

11. Fantus J: The 10% solution to lab profitability. *MLO* 1990;22:33–38.

12. Nelson L: Cost containment: Why not try an idea bank? *MLO* 1983;15:105–108.

13. Gore MJ: The impact of DRGs: II. After five years, coping comes naturally. *MLO* 1988;20:31–35.

14. Becker BL: Cost containment. *MLO* 1983;15:32–46.

19. Marketing

I

T HAS BEEN said, "hospital labs used to let outside testing business find its way to their doors."[1] Many still operate that way. "Lab services are ripe for marketing, and the process will involve lab management deeply in long-range hospital planning."[2]

Marketing promotes maximum use of a hospital's laboratory. An expanded market and full use of laboratory services can make up for monetary deficiencies caused by diagnosis-related group overruns.[3]

Marketing is more than telling clients how reliable your reports will be. Today's clinicians take reliability for granted, so that aspect seldom needs reinforcing. On the other hand, physicians who feel that their pathologists could do a better job of keeping them informed about diagnostic innovations become irritated when they must demand a new service.

"Success demands honesty and wisdom. Honesty is delivering on promises. Wisdom is not promising what you can't deliver."[4]

TARGETS AND SERVICES

There are three strategic marketing goals: (1) do not lose existing clients, (2) get more work from existing clients, and (3) find new clients.[4] The last is the most expensive process.

Laboratories can support their parent organizations' marketing efforts in at least two ways. The first is by helping to increase admissions, a balancing act in which the hospital beds are kept filled, while hospital stays are shortened. The second is to improve the financial status of

156

the institution by striving to continue as a "profit center" instead of converting to "cost center" status. However, success is best measured by satisfying client needs rather than making a profit.

How Laboratories Help to Increase
Hospital Admissions

The importance of fast laboratory service in minimizing inpatient stays is obvious. Physicians, pressured by utilization committees and hospital administrators, expect ancillary services to facilitate inpatient discharges.

Helping to improve the hospital's image in the community is more subtle, and laboratories must cooperate with hospital administration in promoting the total hospital package.

The best hospital sales representatives are clients. Hospitals and laboratories are judged by these consumers from the time of preadmission testing to the moment patients read and try to make sense of their hospital and laboratory bills.

While providing fast, high-quality service is the most important contribution to the hospital's marketing efforts, laboratorians can also help by participating in special educational and promotional activities sponsored by their hospitals. The public is keenly interested in health fairs dealing with topics such as cancer detection, weight control, heart disease, and diabetes. Even small hospital laboratories can sponsor seminars on topics such as coronary risk screening and can offer low-cost laboratory profiles.[5]

Open-house and career-opportunity sessions provide excellent opportunities for the local citizenry to meet hospital personnel.

Bedside Laboratory Testing

Bedside laboratory testing, usually under the direction of the nursing service, is increasing. Usually the hospital laboratory assumes responsibility for quality control of these tests. In some facilities, laboratorians teach patients self-testing, eg, showing diabetics how to monitor their blood sugar levels. When these services are provided grudgingly, nurse and patient customers are ill served.

External Services

The scope and volume of off-site testing will continue to grow. Figures 19.1 and 19.2 list marketing targets and services that can be provided to outpatients and outside facilities.

Remote Phlebotomy Sites

Usually it is best to confine activities at remote phlebotomy sites to specimen collection, but occasionally some on-site testing is indicated.

Physicians' office practices
Physicians' office laboratories
Medical/surgical clinics
Obstetrical/gynecologic practices
Veterinarians
Outpatients
Inpatients (bedside)
Nursing homes
Industries
Legal and social groups
Other hospitals
Wellness programs
Cancer detection programs
Weight control programs

Figure 19.1   Marketing targets.

Physicians' Offices

Because of the influence pathologists have on their active medical staff colleagues, new marketing efforts should target active attending medical staff members first.[6]

Provision of a courier service may be all that a client wants. The timing and frequency of calls is important. At the other end of the service, how quickly are results received by the physicians?

Many spin-offs are possible. For example, Hatfield[7] found that providing a cytology service garnered new physician clients and other kinds of test work while elevating the overall reputation of a small hospital.[7]

Physicians' Office Laboratories

Laboratories can gain business by simply providing quality control materials and office laboratory consulting advice.[8] Belsey and Baer[9] list the following services that may be offered:

manuals for policies and procedures
quality assurance program
proficiency testing
QC materials and interpretation of QC results
equipment maintenance and repair
training of office laboratory staff

```
Phlebotomy
Courier
Specimen collecting stations
Mobile laboratories
Routine/special laboratory tests
Cytology smears
Prenatal screens
Quality control
Business practices
Administrative control
Educational seminars
```

Figure 19.2   Services provided.

assistance with laboratory design and the selection and purchase of equipment and supplies

Arguments over acceptability of preadmission testing done in physicians' office laboratories should be settled amicably, with emphasis on quality of testing, not financial considerations.

Medical Clinics

Clinics and large physician groups often have laboratories that are ripe for takeover by hospital laboratories, especially since quality assurance laws have been extended to include them. Economy of scale would allow much testing within large medical group practices to be performed more economically at hospital laboratories.[6]

Careful analysis of the fiscal aspect and turnaround times is required to provide the swiftest and best service to the clients. Usually a decision must be made as to which tests are performed on site and which ones are transferred to the hospital laboratory. Factors such as courier schedules, computerized reporting, and on-site staffing are considered.

Nursing Homes

Tolin[10] reported that his small hospital laboratory wrested business from reference laboratories by making phlebotomy rounds at nursing homes and staying open for outpatients 24 hours a day.[10] Often other ancillary services such as electrocardiograms, portable x-rays, or inhalational therapy must also be provided.[6]

Other Hospitals

Consolidation of laboratory services of hospitals at different geographic sites can reduce operating expenses while improving their competitive stance in the marketplace.[6] The laboratories of some medical centers have sufficient sophistication to compete with large commercial laboratories in providing esoteric testing, but competition is keen.

Industrial Clients

Among industrial clients, lawn and gardening firms generally desire cholinesterase assays of their employees, battery manufacturers want to check lead levels, and prisons and professional sport teams monitor drug levels of guards, inmates, and athletes. Many large companies require executive and preemployment physical examinations that include some laboratory testing.[6]

Bennett[11] described how he developed a successful drug abuse testing program. Wass and Mohr[12] increased their reference revenue 10% to 15% by providing laboratory services to veterinarians.[12]

Wellness testing, such as cardiac and cancer screening tests, gives laboratories an opportunity to do more than bring in added revenue. It enables them to promote further the quality, expertise, and true value of clinical testing through increased interaction with the public.[13]

PLANS AND STRATEGY

A marketing strategy begins with a needs analysis that focuses on consumer wants. A marketing audit leads to strategy formulation. This usually necessitates a collaborative planning approach in which the laboratory's role is only one segment of a total marketing effort by the organization. A sound strategy includes objectives, programs, implementation, organization, and control.[14]

A needs analysis based principally on formal or informal contact with clients or potential clients should also include information on business trends obtained from such sources as journals, vendors, professional meetings, and seminars.[4] When ambitious marketing efforts are undertaken, it is wise to hire a professional market analyst to prepare a marketing plan and assist in the formulation of a strategy.

Components of a Thorough Marketing Plan

When you have prepared your marketing plan use the following checklist to determine the completeness of your plan:

1. Consumer-oriented situational analysis[4]:
   identification of market segments
   goals and objectives
   analysis of internal operational issues
   development of revenue and expense projections

implementation

evaluation

2. Specific items to be addressed[6]:

special tests or profiles desired

impact of incremental test volume on existing operations

communication support

courier schedules

billing methodology

competitive issues

pricing issues

3. Components of internal operations:

current staffing or equipment needs

projected expenses

specimen acquisition

data handling

problem resolution

report generation

4. Useful tools for surveying customer needs:

questionnaire to active or potential physician clients, nursing homes and other
targets

personal contacts with clients

personal contacts with clients' personnel

personal contacts with laboratory employees:

pathologists

sales reps

managers and supervisors

FINANCIAL ASPECTS

I have mentioned the three marketing goals: keeping current clients, augmenting work referred from these clients, and getting new clients. The first of these goals is by far the most important for two reasons. The marketing costs of landing a new customer are as much as six times those of retaining an old one.[15] And, if old clients cannot be retained, neither will new ones.

While increased use of a laboratory's services may result in overall cost savings, and most hospital laboratories have an excess testing capacity, incremental work loads can play havoc with the scheduling of personnel.[6]

COMPETITION

New projects are rarely undertaken in a vacuum. Competitors can be formidable. A simple process that can be used is the SWOT analytical technique. To perform a SWOT analysis, formulate a list of each of these four factors:

*S*trengths
*W*eaknesses
*O*pportunities
*T*hreats

A brainstorming group will produce the most comprehensive lists, which can be documented on a flip chart. After all ideas have been exhausted, evaluate the importance of each item. A thorough SWOT analysis may prevent an ill-advised endeavor or reveal previously unconsidered opportunities. This analysis will also help when designing a specific marketing program.

LEGAL PITFALLS

Aggressive marketing efforts hold the potential for legal controversy based on federal or state antitrust statutes. Attempts to monopolize, apply unfair methods of competition, or join with competitors to divide geographic service markets can get laboratories into legal trouble. So can kickbacks, bribes, and rebates.[3]

There are tax implications because the policy of the tax laws is that exempt organizations should not have an unfair tax advantage if they engage in activities unrelated to their exempt purpose. The Internal Revenue Service considers a hospital's income from diagnostic tests for nonpatients as prima facie unrelated business income unless an exception to the general rule applies. Therefore, expanded marketing efforts should not be implemented without a review of the likely impact of tax rules.[3]

CLIENT REPRESENTATIVES

"Listen to your sales reps — they're the eyes and ears of your business."[16]

While every laboratorian should be a client representative, some employees shoulder a larger segment of this responsibility. Two of these employees are the in-house client-laboratory coordinator and the external sales representative.

In-House Client-Laboratory Coordinator

The disadvantage of reserving one position for addressing client complaints is that this precludes the other employees from becoming customer conscious. However, having a designated telephone number and a friendly, helpful employee who is thoroughly familiar with the laboratory operation and services can do much for good customer relations.

The duties of this post can be much more comprehensive than simply absorbing gripes. The responsibilities may include reporting test results, quoting prices, dispatching supplies, answering technical questions regarding patient preparation and specimen collection, and clarifying reports or bills.[16]

Functions of Laboratory (or Hospital) Sales Representatives

1. Explain the benefits of the laboratory service to clients.
2. Determine customers' needs.
3. Help develop or improve promotional material, schedules, forms, and newsletters.
4. Handle problems or complaints.
5. Explain new services to customers.
6. Promote the laboratory through open houses, seminars for physicians' office personnel, and speaking engagements.[1]
7. Report on competitors.

For readers who are responsible for planning and managing a hospital sales team, I recommend the book *Managing the Hospital Sales Team* by Williams.[17]

In-house customer service representatives and external sales representatives should have either open invitations or scheduled appearances at staff meetings to discuss client commendations, wants, suggestions, and complaints. At these meetings they should serve as patients' advocates, not hospital or laboratory representatives.

REFERENCES

1. Crane SS: A guide to marketing your laboratory's services. *MLO* 1982;14:41–45.
2. Snook ID Jr: The challenge facing hospitals. In Fitzgibbon R, Statland BE (eds): *DRG Survival Manual for the Clinical Lab*. Oradell, NJ, Medical Economics Books, 1985, pp 17–20.
3. Polk LT: Avoid conflict: Know the legal implications. *Pathologist* 37:8 August 1983;37:546–548.
4. Fantus J: A guide to marketing your lab's services: I. Laying the groundwork. *MLO* 1987;19:39–45.
5. Schmidt SA: A big public service project by a small hospital lab. *MLO* 1988;20:48–51.
6. Portugal B: Strategic planning for outreach laboratory services. *Pathologist* 1983;37:537–540.
7. Hatfield JD: Building outpatient volume through Pap smear testing. *MLO* 1989;21:77–79.
8. Moser E: A support program for physicians' office labs. *MLO* 1989;21:59–62.
9. Belsey R, Baer DM: The technologist's role in quality management of off-site testing: II. *MLO* 1987;19:45–53.
10. Tolin J: Making lab service more accessible to outpatients. *MLO* 1989;21:61–63.
11. Bennett WD: How we marketed drug abuse testing. *MLO* 1989;21:65–72.

12. Wass JA, Mohr R: Guidelines for getting into the veterinary market. *MLO* 1988;20:28–34.

13. Ash K, Urry FM, Smith AW: Wellness testing: New opportunities for clinical labs. *MLO* 1989;21:26–31.

14. White KM: Beginning an overall marketing program in the clinical laboratory. *Hospitals.* 1982;56:104–110.

15. Goldzimer LS: *'I'm first': Your Customer's Message to You.* New York, Rawson Associates, 1989.

16. Fantus J: A guide to marketing your lab's services: II. Launching the sales effort. *MLO* 1987;19:57–62.

17. Williams RC: *Managing the Hospital Sales Team.* Chicago, American Hospital Publishing Inc, 1988.

20. Quality Assurance

T HE DANGER "LIES in a naive and atheoretical belief, rampant today in the orgy of measurement, that the assessment and publication of performance data will somehow induce otherwise indolent care givers to improve the level of their care and efficiency."[1] Quality assurance (QA) is a planned and systematic process for monitoring and evaluating the quality and appropriateness of patient care. This care must be consistent with standards established by medical, nursing, and departmental professionals, as well as by regulatory or accrediting agencies.

QA is defined by the JCAHO as "the degree to which patient-care services increase the probability of desired patient outcomes and reduce the probability of undesired outcomes, given the current state of knowledge."[2] In the clinical laboratory, JCAHO inspectors look for a laboratory's ability to define a QA problem, propose changes, implement action, and monitor follow-up.[3]

ESSENTIALS OF QA: STRUCTURE-PROCESS-OUTCOME

The *structure* consists of policies, rules, regulations, standards of operations, and credentials that provide guidelines on how quality care is to be provided.

The *process* describes how what is expressed in these documents is carried out.

The *outcomes* describe results, such as timely and accurate reports or the restoration of depleted blood volume.

STATISTICAL *V* HUMANISTIC QA

There are four characteristics of quality care. It is (1) safe, (2) appropriate, (3) timely, and (4) sensitive. Most QA programs described in the medical and laboratory literature seem to assign a low priority to the sensitivity characteristic. I recently sat in on a JCAHO medical inspector's summation at our hospital. Not once did he use the word "patient," "client," "consumer," or "customer".

Laboratory approaches to QA are largely extensions of quality control, with emphasis on data accumulation and statistical analysis rather than improved client satisfaction. "Even the best of process and product measures lead to suboptimization unless combined with measures of customer satisfaction."[4] QA coordinators are being appointed in droves, but they are just more paper shufflers who spend most of their time in offices isolated from clients.

Berwick[1] put it succinctly and correctly when he wrote that "too much effort goes into looking for better tools of inspection in the search for outliers, thus applying the 'Theory of Bad Apples'." As a result, minimal standards quickly become ceilings, and overall quality plateaus at low levels.

QA as presently practiced relies principally on inspection and statistical analysis, disregarding what Japanese business experts keep telling us — that the "Theory of Continuous Improvement" *(kaizen)* is vastly superior to this old hunt-and-peck system. Kaizen focuses on intense education rather than monitoring. It involves every employee, not just a select group. It prevents rather than corrects deficiencies. It is proactive, not reactive. Kinkus and McMann[3] also emphasize the importance of staff education in any lab QA program.

We tend to monitor the things that are easiest to monitor and that are easily expressed in numbers, the "hard data" we laboratorians worship. When improperly administered, QA can actually lower rather than improve client satisfaction. Take phlebotomists, for example. If the emphasis is on turnaround time, and the only other indicators are obtaining sufficient blood volume and putting it into the right tubes, how does that affect the interpersonal relationships between hurried phlebotomists and their patient clients?

It is unfortunate that QA is being pushed so vigorously at a time when there is a drive to lower costs. Nursing services and laboratories are experiencing reductions in force, while clerks and bean counters proliferate. Nurses leave critical care units for less stressful jobs in QA, utilization review, and related activities. If a laboratory position must be eliminated, who goes — the educational coordinator or the QA coordinator? Which job would a practitioner of kaizen eliminate?

The step beyond QA is total quality management, a proactive approach based principally on client expectations, and depending largely on intensive training to prevent problems, not on variances, as determined by indicator or monitoring systems. Some industrial companies, such as 3M Corporation, already have these in place.[5]

THE COLLEGE OF AMERICAN PATHOLOGISTS

The College of American Pathologists (CAP) has for many years provided programs that assist laboratories in their quality control and quality assurance activities. These programs include laboratory accreditation, surveys, quality assurance service, work load recording method, and, more recently "Q-probe," which is an interlaboratory quality improvement program encompassing a broad spectrum of criteria such as nosocomial infection rates, turnaround times, surgical pathology consultations, and low-quality specimens.[6,7]

The Three Activity Areas of Laboratory QA

1. Activities within the laboratory to ensure accuracy, precision and speed. This is largely quality control.
2. Interactions between the ordering physician and the laboratory. These include ease of requesting service, turnaround times, and charting of results—the beginning and end of the work flow.
3. Use and abuse of laboratory services by physicians. This involves monitoring stat testing and prescribing the appropriate tests by the physicians, ie, laboratory utilization.

THE TEN-STEP PROCESS OF THE JCAHO

Most laboratory QA programs are patterned after JCAHO guidelines.[2] Following is a description of this ten-step process.

1. Assign Responsibility

Every employee strives to provide quality service, but QA coordinators and QA committees are usually responsible for monitoring and evaluating the process, aided and supported by the laboratory management team.

2. Delineate Scope of Care

The scope of a service includes all of the major diagnostic and product services as described in laboratory user manuals.

3. Identify Important Aspects of Care

This is a critical step. Topics selected are usually (1) high risk (eg, blood component therapy), (2) high volume (eg, biochemical profiles), (3) problem prone (eg, 24-hour urine studies), (4) expensive (eg, endocrine studies), or (5) invasive (eg, fine needle aspirates).[8]

Selection of problem areas is facilitated by obtaining feedback from a variety of sources (Figure 20.1).

4. Identify Indicators

Once a procedure is selected, a tactical approach is constructed. The study may be directed at the medical aspect, eg, how tests are ordered, reported, and

Incident reports

Committee reports
  Laboratory utilization
  Hospital utilization
  Transfusion
  Infection control
  Medical records
  Education

Surveys
  Patients
  Physicians
  Other departments
    Nursing service
    Finance
    Emergency room
    Operating suite
    Medical records
    Materials management
    Human resources
    Admission office
    Outpatient department

Coordinators or staff specialists
  Quality assurance
  Safety
  Laboratory information service
  Sales representatives

Productivity reports
  CAP work load
  Institutional financial reports

Credential Reviews

Figure 20.1   Sources used to identify problems.

interpreted. It may focus on technical aspects, eg, quality control. It may be administrative, eg, incident reports and user satisfaction surveys.[9]

After the direction has been decided on, appropriate indicators must be formulated. An indicator is a well-defined variable related to the structure, process, or outcome of care. Indicators should be objective and measurable. A list of typical laboratory indicators is shown in Figure 20.2.

There are two kinds of indicators: sentinal event indicators and comparative rate indicators. Sentinal event indicators identify rare but serious outcomes, eg, transfusion reaction due to mismatched blood. Comparative rate indicators deal with events that require review of cases when the rate of the event exceeds or falls below an established threshold or when significant variance over time is identi-

```
Quality control
Productivity
Identity of patients and specimens
Specimen rejection
Specimen preparation
Turnaround time
Reporting of "panic values"
Blood component utilization
Infection control and safety
Laboratory utilization
Client satisfaction
```

Figure 20.2 Typical laboratory QA indicators.

fied. A high incidence of single blood cultures or a low incidence of posttransfusion hemoglobin determinations would raise concern.

In addition to identifying the type of indicator and describing the indicator population, investigators document the rationale (why the indicator is useful) and the indicator logic (data elements and data sources), eg, the start and completion of phlebotomy rounds (data); and laboratory section logs (data source).

5. Establish Thresholds for Evaluations

Each structure indicator (eg, maintenance log), process indicator (eg, turnaround time), and outcome indicator (eg, hemoglobin change after transfusion) must have a threshold.[9] These thresholds can be based on clinical and QA publications, or on the experience of the laboratory staff.

Criteria are needed to define the thresholds precisely. For example, an indicator dealing with laboratory utilization requires criteria to delineate excessive or inappropriate test use.[10] In designing criteria, test order priorities must be considered. For example, turnaround times for routine, urgent, and stat orders are usually different.

6. Collect and Organize Data

Monitoring may be retrospective or concurrent. The former consists of review of records or incident reports. Concurrent studies comprise ongoing observations.

This data collection and organization may be done by a QA coordinator or a QA committee. Data sources include proficiency testing results,[3] performance appraisals, medical charts, laboratory logs, quality control records, and data from focused studies such as the "Q-probes" of the CAP.[11] Sharp[8] described a statistically valid method of randomly selecting patients' charts for monitoring laboratory utilization. The tests or orders most frequently audited by his committee were standing orders for laboratory work, high-cost tests, esoteric tests, and invasive tests.

Periodic audits review compliance with specific policies and evaluate the performance of problem-prone tests, instruments, and people.

QA Charts Are Useful

Charts list data month by month and for the year. Equipment logs document downtime; investigation and follow-up forms record results of proficiency surveys. Complaints and commendations should all be documented. LIS provides statistical data on test volumes, percentage of stat orders, turnaround times, and much more.

Problem-Solving Forms

Most QA programs use special problem-solving forms. These consist of descriptions of what went wrong, how it was handled, and how it can be prevented.

7. Evaluate Care

To evaluate care, demonstrated performance is compared with the desired indicator and threshold.[9] The plan should include a description of excluding factors. These may be factors over which no one has control or the control may be in the hands of people outside the laboratory. For example, only one blood culture may have been performed because a patient died before other specimens were obtained; a prolonged power failure may have delayed the turnaround time.

8. Take Action to Solve Problems

Determine the causes of variances such as lack of knowledge or training, poor motivation, lack of adequate equipment or supplies, insufficient or incompetent personnel.

This may lead to an investigation of soft spots in personnel selection, orientation, training, and retention.

9. Assess the Actions and Document Improvement

Follow-up is usually carried out by coordinators or committees. Monthly QA reports should be discussed at department meetings.

10. Communicate Relevant Information

Implementation and documentation are not enough, the best QA programs are educational, not coercive or punitive. To maximize the educational benefits, problems and solutions should receive widespread dissemination. This is best achieved by discussions at staff meetings.

The organizational QA committee and the hospital executives must be kept informed and their support solicited.

PATHOLOGIC ANATOMY

Cowan[12] described a comprehensive pathologic anatomy system of QA centered around defined standards, performance monitors, peer review, technical and clerical review, documented action to define and remedy problems, reporting, and coherence with institutional programs. His program is conveniently divided into professional performance and system operations. As an example, each surgical pathology case is evaluated for correctness and wording of diagnosis, timeliness of report, adequacy of tissue sampling, and quality of histologic preparations.

SUCCESS STORIES

Most QA articles relate strategy and tactics. Success is usually expressed in global comments and without much mention of cost-benefit ratios, or even significant positive results. Kinkus and McMann[3] reported that their longstanding problem of sharing urine specimens by two laboratory sections was eliminated. Does it really take a QA program to detect and solve such a simple problem of coordination?

REFERENCES

1. Berwick DM: Continuous improvement as an ideal in health care. *N Engl J Med* 1989;320:53–56.
2. *Medical Staff Monitoring and Evaluation: Departmental Review.* Chicago, Joint Commission on Accreditation of Healthcare Organizations, 1985–1989.
3. Kinkus CA, McMann NW: A sweeping QA program for a large hospital lab. *MLO* 1990;22:31–35.
4. Davidow WB, Uttal B: *Total Customer Service: The Ultimate Weapon.* New York, Harper & Row, 1989.
5. Melum MM, Sinioris M: The next generation of health care quality. *Hospitals* 1989;63:80.
6. *Standards for Laboratory Accreditation.* Northfield, IL, College of American Pathologists, 1987.
7. Schifman RB: Infection control serves as quality assurance model. *CAP Today* 1988;2:12.
8. Sharp JW: Implementing hospitalwide laboratory QA. *MLO* 1989;21:35–38.
9. Berte LM: Growing into laboratory quality assurance. *MLO* 1990;22:24–29.

10. Parsek JD: Letter to Editor. *Nurs Manage* 1989;20:13–14.

11. *Q-Probes*. Northfield, IL, College Of American Pathologists, 1989.

12. Cowan DF: Quality assurance in anatomic pathology. *Arch Pathol Lab Med* 1990;114:29–134.

21. Leaders in the Client-Oriented Laboratory

THE CHALLENGE IS simple. Satisfy clients or step aside for someone who will. Throughout this book we have detailed what employers must do to improve client service. The implementation process is the responsibility of managers at all levels. In this final chapter we focus on managerial competencies and characteristics essential in developing a customer-oriented work ethic.

CHANGING A CULTURE IS NOT EASY

Developing a customer-oriented culture is difficult and slow. It is much harder than achieving leadership in technology, cost containment, or quality control. Building dedication to service may take several years.[1] One sign of success is when employees start concentrating on pleasing clients more than on pleasing bosses or meeting the mandates of accrediting agencies.

Employees model their values on those of their leaders. Laboratory leaders must be change leaders, capable of overcoming many obstacles, the most difficult of which are human. Leaders must be patient, persistent, and consistent.[2]

Bureaucratic leadership will not do. When employees are guided only by policies, rules and regulations, bureaucratic leadership with all its red tape and road blocks, service will be sabotaged.

"Strong leadership ensures that service to the customer doesn't lose out to the bean counters."[1]

173

IMPROVED CLIENT SERVICE ALWAYS INVOLVES CHANGE

Leaders must know precisely what their clients want, and how well these wants are being met. Too often managers make changes based on the managers' perceptions of what is best for the clients, without bothering to ask the clients. Too often, the absence of formal complaints is interpreted as being indicative of good service.

"Change 'is a vehicle' that needs a driver. The driver must have a 'take-charge-can-do' attitude."[2]

Each of the six basic functions of management — planning, staffing, organizing, coordinating, directing, and controlling — must be executed expertly. In the client-oriented laboratory, directing and controlling are muted in favor of coaching, training, cheerleading, encouraging innovation, and fostering responsibility.

The basic supervisory skills of motivating, teaching, communicating, decision making, managing time, delegating, and developing careers are all essential.

Ultimately, laboratory leaders must do more than proclaim superior client service. Unless they back these proclamations with actions, their customers and their employees will view the effort as just another transient public relations gimmick.

Customer-oriented leaders become personally involved in pleasing clients, always talk about customers, tell stories of exceptional service, and publicize the compliments earned by their teammates. They put their values into action by treating employees as they want employees to treat customers.[1]

CREATE YOUR OWN TEAM OF EXPERTS

Change specialists recognize and acknowledge their personal limitations. They supplement their own expertise with that of others. For example, their competencies may include the ability to select and train the right people, to coach effectively, and to motivate, but they may lack innovativeness, marketing skill, or medical diagnostic expertise.

Innovators and "entrepreneurs" are "skilled at integrating trends and data into concepts and plans, solving problems in new ways, identifying possibilities, seizing opportunities, searching for new and better ways of doing things, selling concepts, sensing obstacles, and knowing tricks of getting special resources."[2]

Professional and technical experts possess special knowledge and skill, use state of the art techniques, and have a working knowledge of statistics and data processing.[2]

THE IMPORTANCE OF CONTINUOUS IMPROVEMENT TO EVERY PROVIDER

What satisfies customers today may not satisfy them tomorrow. The challenge leaders face is to maintain competitiveness through creative approaches to work assignments that maximize human and machine resources.[3]

As competition increases, so does the need for continuous improvement. This is achieved only when policies, training, and relationships inspire every employee to strive for service improvement.[4]

Leaders make customer service everyone's business. They encourage each employee to feel and act as if he or she owns the unit.[1] Only by drawing on the combined brain power of all its employees can a department provide the best service.

PROVIDING SUPPORT TO EMPLOYEES

Managers must view workers more as equal partners than as silent followers. Genuine cooperation requires that employees contribute to the perception and definition of problems as well as to their solution.[5]

Support must not be manipulative under the guise of "participative management." According to Katzman,[6] what is termed participative management is often a placebo that gives workers the trappings of decision-making power. The workers soon realize that their quality circles, problem-solving groups, and committees represent only new versions of management's familiar old attempts to increase commitment, and that they are allowed to make only those decisions that do not infringe on the prerogatives of the members of the executive suite.[6]

BARRIERS TO CHANGE

Too often there is not only a lack of support, but even managerial roadblocks that prevent employees from doing their jobs. Support comes in the form of "user-friendly" policies and rules, from treating employees as equals, from providing the necessary supplies and equipment, from minimizing work hazards, and from helping employees to develop technical and professional expertise.

Support also includes large doses of training and education. Japanese companies give their employees three to four times more training than do their American counterparts.[7]

Leaders must be able to overcome many other human and organizational barriers to change. They must be patient, persistent, and consistent.

All processes generate some variances that adversely affect service, and any sociotechnical system is only as good as management's ability to control these variances.[4] One example is the employee whose behavior is adversely affecting customer relations.

The Bad Apples

Client service can suffer grievously if just one or two employees do not perform up to client expectations. Extensive customer feedback is necessary to detect all of these bad apples. Some of these "outliers" are negativists, some are chronic complainers, and others just do not give a hoot about the people being served. It is up to leaders to ferret out these individuals and take quick action. The appropriate action may be to remove them from client contact, to change their behavior, or to get rid of them.

It is not easy to dispose of an employee whose quality and quantity of work meets your performance standards but who neglects or irritates clients. Blood collectors may be very capable phlebotomists, but if they argue with coworkers in the presence of patients, they threaten your program. If a nurse in a blood donor center turns away a potential donor because he or she arrived 5 minutes late, that nurse is also undermining a program. If a pathologist cancels many of his staff meetings or lectures to work on his personal research project, he is neglecting his clients.

Summary

Following is a list of the most important points I have discussed:

All service providers must know who their customers are: patients, patients' families, visitors, attending physicians, nurses, other hospital departments, committees, and special staff members. Fellow employees, students, and superiors are also recipients of laboratory services (Chapter 1).

Formal and informal client feedback systems must be used frequently to monitor customer satisfaction (Chapter 1).

Client awareness is more difficult for laboratory employees because, for the most part, the customer is invisible (Chapter 1).

Client satisfaction is a process, not a program (Chapter 2).

The laboratory mission statement should feature client satisfaction (Chapter 2).

In the client-oriented laboratory, client satisfaction is everyone's business (Chapter 2).

Group participation is facilitated through team building, quality circles, and other employee participation groups (Chapters 3 through 6).

The importance of continuous training and education cannot be overemphasized. This training begins with a comprehensive indoctrination program for new employees (Chapters 3 and 9).

Like customer service elsewhere, providers must expect and accommodate difficult clients. Special training in coping with these customers should be provided to all laboratory workers, especially those who have frequent customer contact (Chapters 3 and 15).

Client orientation must be reinforced through position descriptions, work standards, performance reviews, and reward systems (Chapters 7 and 10).

The selection process for new employees should focus on identifying candidates who have a client-oriented attitude (Chapter 8).

All forms of communication are important, but none is more critical than person-to-person contacts (Chapters 11 through 13).

Training in telephone courtesy is a must (Chapter 12).

Achieving change is best accomplished by an egalitarian approach, with full participation by all members of the laboratory staff (Chapter 14).

Changes in behavioral norms occur only when people accept the fact that new norms are needed (Chapter 14).

Laboratory leaders must preach client satisfaction and consistently model exemplary behavior (Chapter 16).

Improved retention of personnel is an essential component of any customer-service program (Chapter 16).

Customers who pay for the cost of laboratory service expect improved productivity and cost containment. (Chapters 17 and 18).

Marketing should be based primarily on meeting customer expectations. This can be effective only when these expectations are known (Chapter 19).

Members of the client-oriented laboratory spend more time responding to the wants of customers than to the demands of superiors or accrediting agencies (Chapter 20).

Quality assurance programs that do not give client satisfaction the highest priority must be converted into total quality management programs that do (Chapter 20).

Customer satisfaction is reflected in how employees are treated (Chapter 21).

Employees must be encouraged to innovate, to take calculated risks, and not to be overly concerned with judgmental mistakes, unless the mistakes concern patients' test results or a therapeutic blood component (Chapter 21).

One or two bad performers can wreak havoc with the best of programs. Employees who will not, or who cannot change, must be transferred to less sensitive posts or must be separated (Chapter 21).

REFERENCES

1. Davidow WH, Uttal B: *Total Customer Service: The Ultimate Weapon.* New York, Harper & Row, 1989.

2. Dalziel MM, Schoonover SC: *Changing Ways: A Practical Tool for Implementing Change Within Organizations.* New York, AMACOM Book Division, 1988.

3. Schein E: Organizational Culture. *Am Psychologist* 1990;45:109.

4. Greenwood F, Kobu B: Management modifications. *SAM Adv Manage* 1990; 55:33.

5. Levitan S, Johnson C: Labor and management: The illusion of cooperation. *Harvard Bus Rev* 1983;000:8–16.

6. Katzman MS: US labor policy and its implications for South Korea. *SAM Adv Manage J* 1990; 55:9–13.

7. Matsushita K, quoted in Greenwood F, Kobu B: Management modifications. *SAM Adv Manage J* 1990;55:30–33.

Index

Numbers in **boldface** refer to pages on which figures appear.

C

Capital budget, 147, 149–150
CAP units/worked hours, **151**
Career-opportunity session, 157
Cash budget, 147
Cause-and-effect diagram, 40, **41**
Celebrations, 20, 70
Chairperson, for quality circle, 13
Change
  barriers to, 175
  checklist, 109, **110**
  continuous need for, 174–175
  garnering support for, 113–114, **113**
  implementation of, 114–115
  imposed, adjusting to, 118
  instrument selection, 112–113
  management's role in, 173–176
  overcoming resistance to, 115–118
  plans and strategies for, 109
  preparing for, 108–110
  procedural, 13–14
  reviewing previous changes, 109
  structural, 13–14
  training program for, 115
  written proposal for, 110–112
Charge/test, 150
Cheerleading, 174
Chronic complainer, 128–129, 175
Client. *See* Customer
Coaching process, 133–134, 174
College of American Pathologists: quality assurance programs, 166–167
Commendation, 77, 170
  written, 106–107
Commendation form, 5
Comment card, 73, 121
Committee report, 168
  as feedback source, 5
Communication, 16, 20–22, 50, 139, 174. *See also* Telephone etiquette
  about impending changes, 117–118
  body language, 89–92
  listening skill, 87–88
  oral, 83–92, 101
  in performance appraisal, 78, **79**

providers as senders, 83
providers as receivers, 86
psychological barriers to, 85–86
semantic barriers to, 85
written. *See* Written communication
Competition between laboratories, 161–162
Competitive advantage, 108
Complainer, 120–129
  chronic, 128–129, 175
  hostile, 125–127
Complaint, 5, 14, 120–129, 170
  by angry customer, 124–125
  channels for registering, 121
  discussion by employee participating groups, 27
  documentation of, 15
  by employee, 127–128
  by hostile complainer, 125–127
  in-house client-laboratory coordinator, 162
  methods of handling, 121
  in performance appraisal, 77
  problem-solving letter, 106
  reasons for, 120–121
  steps in dealing with, 122–123, **124–125**
  telephone calls, 98–99
Complaint form, 4, 5, **6–7**
Computerization, 145, 152
Computer language, 85
Concealment, signs of, 91
Confidence, signs of, 92
Confrontational skills, 20
Consensus, in brainstorming, 44–45
Continuous improvement. *See* Change
Cost/benefit analysis, 40
Cost/test, 150
Cost containment, 27, 146–155
  equipment costs, 153
  quality-control costs, 153
  ratios to focus on problems, 151, **152**
  reagent costs, 152
  reference laboratory fees, 153
  staff budget reductions, 151–152

consolidation of laboratory services, 160
orientation program, 63–65
sales representative, 157
Hostile complainer, 125–127
Hybrid generalist-specialist, 20

I

Impatience, signs of, 91
Improvement. *See also* Change
theory of continuous improvement, 10
Incident report, 14–15, 17, 121, 168–169
Income statement, 147
Indicator
comparative rate, 168
sentinal event, 168
Indirect costs, 149
Indirect costs/net sales, **152**
Indoctrination program. *See* Orientation program
Industrial client, 160
Inflammatory words, **125**
Infrastructure, 12–13
barriers to productivity, 139–140
Initiative, employee, 50
Innovation, encouragement of, 144, 174
Input time, decreases in, 142–143
In-service educational program, 17–22
changing employee behavior with, 18–20
for customer contact agents, 21–22
training for quality circles, 32
Instrumentation, 145. *See also* Equipment acquisition
Interdepartmental relationships, 47
Internal customer, 1–2
Interrelationship standards, 50
Interview
exit, 130–131
job candidate. *See* Job candidate interview

performance appraisal, 73–76
Intralaboratory newsletter, 16
Intuition, 36
Inventory control, 30, 154
IPC technique, 44

J

Jargon, 85, 104–105
JCAHO. *See* Joint Commission on Accreditation of Healthcare Organizations
Jigsaw puzzle fallacy, 37
Job candidate interview
closing of, 58–59
first impression in, 58
handling sensitive issues in, 58
preparation checklist for, 57
questions asked in, 55–57
signs of turnover susceptibility, 132, **132–133**
untruthful candidate, 58
Job description. *See* Position description
Job offer, 61
Job satisfaction, 20
Joint Commission on Accreditation of Healthcare Organizations (JCAHO), 13
quality assurance guidelines, 167–171
Judgment in problem solving, 36
suspended, 40–41

K

Kaizen, 166

L

Laboratory information service specialist, 68
Laboratory log, 169

objectives of, 62–63
"show and tell time", 66
Output standards, 141
Output time, decreases in, 143

P

Pareto chart, 40, **42**
Parking, 140
Participative management, 175
Part-time employee, 152
PAS approach to written communication, 106
Pathologic anatomy; quality assurance, 171
Patient, as customer, 1–2
Patient care, evaluation of, 170
Patient self-testing, 157
Patients' representative, 5, 13, 121
Payable test, 150
Pay-for-performance system, 14
Payroll data, 147
Payroll insert, 18
Peer review organization, 13
People relationships, description of, 47–48
Percent productivity, **151**
Performance appraisal, 14–15, 72–82, 169
  discussion of future, 78–81
  discussion of past, 77
  reverse of roles, 8, 72, 81–82
  salary discussion, 73, 76
  steps in, 76–81
  updating position description, 76–77
Performance appraisal form, 77
Performance appraisal interview, 73–76
Performance criteria, 48
Performance levels, 49–50
Performance monitoring, 15
Performance rating system, 14–15
Performance standards, 46, 49–53
  compliance, 50

customer-oriented, 52–53
customer-oriented words, 52
interrelationship, 50
quality assurance words, 52
quantifying, 51–52
setting levels of, 49–50
task, 51
temperament, 50
Personnel. *See* Employee
Persuasion, 18–19
Phlebotomist
  customer-oriented performance standards for, 53
  employee participating groups, 26–27
  in-service programs for, 18
  retention of, 22
Phlebotomy site, remote, 157
Physician, as customer, 1, 3
Physicians' office laboratory, 28
  as marketing target, 158–159
Planning, 30
  group, 19
  strategic, 11–12
Planning session following performance review, 73
Policy making, 30
Position description, 14
  people relationships, 47–48
  qualifications, 47
  responsibilities, duties, and tasks, 48–49
  standards, work 46, 49–51
  summary statement, 46–47
  updating of, 76–77
  verbs for, 48–49
Position purpose. *See* Position summary
Position summary, 46–47
Power, signs of, 92
Praise, 69, 134
Praise-criticism ratio, 69
Preadmission testing, 159
Precision, employee, 51
Preemployment tests, 55
Presentation of proposal, 112

Proactive strategy, to avert resignation, 135
Problem solving, 20, 170, 175
  bias in, 40
  brainstorming, 40–42
  confirmation trap in, 40
  developing active plan, 39
  evaluating alternatives, 38–39
  follow-up of, 39
  generating alternatives, 38
  getting and interpreting facts, 37–38
  by quality circle, 33
  salami approach to, 39
  seeking consensus, 44–45
  stating objectives in, 38–39
  steps to, 37–39
  tools in, 40
  traps in, 40
  troubleshooting alternatives, 39
Problem-solving forms, 170
Problem-solving group, 36
  charge to, 36–37
Problem-solving letter, 106
Productivity
  definition of, 138
  extrinsic barriers to, 139–140
  improvement of, 138–145, 152
  intrinsic barriers to, 140–141
  investigation of productivity problem, 141–142
  measurement of, 141
  strategic objectives, 139
  ways to increase, 142–145
Productivity/FTE hour, **151**
Productivity norms, 140–141, 144
Productivity rate, 51
Productivity report, 168
Profanity, 127
Proficiency test, 158, 169–170
Promotion, 15
Proposal, written. *See* Written proposal
Prospective payment, 146
Prospective pricing, 150
Psychographic information, 11, **12**
Punctuality, employee, 50

Purchasing practices, 152, 154
Put-down in communication, 88, **89**

Q

QA. *See* Quality assurance
QC. *See* Quality circle
Q-probe, 167, 169
Qualifications of candidates, description of, 47
Quality assurance (QA), 158–159
  CAP program, 166–167
  collecting and organizing data, 169–170
  educational aspects of, 170
  evaluation of patient care, 170
  follow-up on, 170
  identifying important aspects of care, 167, **168**
  indentifying indicators, 167–169, **169**
  JCAHO guidelines, 167–171
  pathologic anatomy system of, 171
  problem-solving, 170
  statistical *v.* humanistic, 165–166
  structure-process-outcome, 165
  success of, 171
  thresholds for evaluations, 169
Quality assurance (QA) chart, 170
Quality assurance (QA) committee, 167, 169, 171. *See also* Quality circle
Quality assurance (QA) coordinator, 68, 167, 169
Quality assurance (QA) words, 52
Quality circle (QC), 20, 26, 29–34, 73, 175
  chairperson of, 13
  definition of, 29–31
  facilitators of, 31–32
  follow-up of, 33–34
  incentives to participate in, 30–31
  leaders of, 31–32
  measuring results of, 33
  meeting agenda, 32–33

V

Vacation schedule, 152
Variable cost/test, **151**
Verbal communication. *See* Oral
    communication
Verbs, in position description, 48–49
Vestibule training, 68
Videotape, educational, 18
Voice mail, 95
Voice quality, 94
"Volcano" person, 126–127
Volunteer, 152

W

Weekend shift, 13
Weight control program, 158
Welcome, letter of, 64
Wellness program, 158, 160
Work flow pattern, 30, 141–142
Work habits, 50
Work load, 140, 143
Workload Reporting System, 141

Workplace signs, 92
Workshop. *See* In-service educational
    program; Training program
Work standards. *See* Performance
    standards
Work station rotation, 83
Written apology, 107
Written commendation, 106–107
Written communication, 101–107
    client consideration in, 102
    editing of, 104–105
    gender-inclusive language in, 104,
        104
    letter, memo, and report writing,
        102–105
    letter *v.* memo, 102
    readability, improving, 102–105
    redundant expressions, **106**
    rewriting, 103–104
    rough draft, 102–103
Written proposal, 110–112
    appendices to, 112
    cover letter for, 112
    format for, 110, **111**
Written reprimand, 107